Feeling Fat, Fuzzy, or Frazzled?

Also by Richard Shames, MD,
and Karilee Shames, PhD, RN

Thyroid Power: Ten Steps to Total Health

Feeling Fat, Fuzzy, or Frazzled?

A 3-STEP PROGRAM TO:

- Beat Hormone Havoc
- Restore Thyroid, Adrenal, and Reproductive Balance
- Feel Better Fast!

Richard Shames, MD

Karilee Shames, PhD, RN

HUDSON
STREET
PRESS

HUDSON STREET PRESS
Published by Penguin Group
Penguin Group (USA) Inc., 375 Hudson Street, New York, New York 10014, U.S.A.
Penguin Group (Canada), 10 Alcorn Avenue, Toronto, Ontario, Canada M4V 3B2
(a division of Pearson Penguin Canada Inc.)
Penguin Books Ltd, 80 Strand, London WC2R 0RL, England
Penguin Ireland, 25 St Stephen's Green, Dublin 2, Ireland (a division of Penguin Books Ltd)
Penguin Group (Australia), 250 Camberwell Road, Camberwell, Victoria 3124, Australia
(a division of Pearson Australia Group Pty Ltd)
Penguin Books India Pvt Ltd, 11 Community Centre, Panchsheel Park,
New Delhi – 110 017, India
Penguin Books (NZ), cnr Airborne and Rosedale Roads, Albany, Auckland 1310,
New Zealand (a division of Pearson New Zealand Ltd)
Penguin Books (South Africa) (Pty) Ltd, 24 Sturdee Avenue, Rosebank,
Johannesburg 2196, South Africa

Penguin Books Ltd, Registered Offices: 80 Strand, London WC2R 0RL, England

First published by Hudson Street Press, a member of Penguin Group (USA) Inc.

First Printing, July 2005
10 9 8 7 6 5 4 3 2 1

REGISTERED TRADEMARK—MARCA REGISTRADA

HUDSON
STREET
PRESS

CIP data is available.
ISBN 1-59463-002-X (alk. paper)

Printed in the United States of America
Set in Janson Text with Futura
Designed by Daniel Lagin

PUBLISHER'S NOTE
Neither the publisher nor the authors intend for the information provided in this book to be construed as engaging in rendering professional advice or services to the individual reader. The resources, ideas, procedures, and suggestions contained in this book are not intended as a substitute for consulting with your physician. Consultation with your physician is advised. The publisher and authors are not responsible for your specific health or allergy needs that may require medical supervision, for any adverse reactions to the products, services, or procedures contained or referred to in this book, or for any loss or damage arising or allegedly arising from any information or suggestion in this book. While the authors have made every effort to provide accurate telephone numbers, Internet and mailing addresses, and other product information at the time of publication, neither the publisher nor the authors assume any responsibility for errors, or for changes that occur after publication.

Many of the products mentioned in this book may be ordered from www.FeelingFFF.com or by calling 866-468-4979. See Appendix for more detailed information.

This book is printed on acid-free paper. ∞

We dedicate this book to our dear friend Michael Jakovich, who made us laugh so much and left us all too soon. We seek to help others in your honor. Be at peace.

This project has been inspired by the years of heartfelt input from patients in our practice. Your observations and honesty have guided us toward creative solutions to the problems that plague so many others.

We thank you from the bottom of our hearts for your courage, commitment, and humor. It is our honor and pleasure to dedicate this work to the growing movement toward better hormone balance and consumer empowerment.

ACKNOWLEDGMENTS

We are grateful to our three children, who have nobly endured the ups and downs of the parental coauthoring process as we once again tangled over ideas and wording:

- Gabe, for bravely living with us as the last child left at home, and for your inspiration as you patiently write your own project.
- Gigi, for your gentle support and endless mix of Buddhist and college humor. Best wishes in your study of acupuncture.
- Shauna, for caring so much about the world, and for doing your best always to make it better. Good luck in teaching and grad school.

We also offer our deepest appreciation to Faith Hamlin of Sanford J. Greenburger Associates, our amazing agent, for her diligent focus in helping us shed new light on persistent health issues.

Our gratitude extends also to our delightful and articulate editor Laureen Rowland, who has guided this project with an informed sensitivity and a masterly vision of what readers truly need from today's health-care providers. Also we give appreciation for Brant Janeway and his marketing and publicity team at Penguin, for helping to launch this book.

We deeply thank Anne McCombs, DO, an especially knowledgeable and generous practitioner in Kirkland, Washington; Ellen Cutler, MD, of Bioset Clinic/Institute in Mill Valley, California; Harold Kristal, DDS, and James Haig, NC, of the Metabolic Nutrition Center in San Rafael, California; as well as Peggy Wolff, MS, APRN, HNC, for her loving guidance as Holistic Nurse and environmental health consultant. (See Resources for all listed.) Special appreciation to Mary Shomon, inspiring patient advocate, author, and Web master. Love to Lynn Larkin and Trinity Whittaker for such great support!

Richard wishes to particularly acknowledge those practitioners who have offered additional understanding of key health issues.

- This includes his colleagues in the San Francisco–area NutriMedicine Doctors Group for providing a forum for bold new ideas.
- Much appreciation to the hardworking practitioners and staff at the Preventive Medicine Center of Marin, where Dr. Shames sees his patients. Special thanks to Judy Lane, Nurse Practitioner par excellence, for her female hormone expertise.
- He also appreciates the tremendous support of several savvy laboratory researchers, including Dr. David Zava of ZRT Labs, Dr. Edward Winger of IDL Labs, Dr. Elias Ilyia of Diagnos-Techs Lab, and the many others who daily serve as pioneers for better diagnosis of subtle health concerns.
- And to Karilee, a gifted practitioner and healer, whose way with words is matched only by her divine goodwill, especially to me.

Karilee wishes to acknowledge those who have enriched her journey.

- She offers her deepest appreciation to her father, Jack Feibus, for his excellent example of perseverance in the face of adversity and for his great sense of humor, which she hopes she inherited.
- And her mom, Gloria Ingraham, for her eternal strength and willingness to learn and grow.
- She thanks her cousin Sherry Deutsch for always being a source of friendship and laughter, her "cuz" and best friend.
- She sends regards to the faculty of the Christine E. Lynn College of Nursing at Florida Atlantic University in Boca Raton, Florida, where her creative ideas were encouraged to flourish under the excellent guidance of Dean Anne Boykin.
- And to Rich, her wonderful partner, who blesses her life with love and laughter.

CONTENTS

COMING BACK TO LIFE: FACING THE GROWING CHALLENGE OF HORMONE HAVOC

Gland imbalance is largely an unsuspected illness.
Even when suspected, it is frequently undiagnosed.
When it is diagnosed, it often goes untreated.
When it is treated, it is seldom treated optimally.

When Jackie* walked into our office, we hardly recognized her. Ten years earlier, at age thirty-two, she had been a vital, attractive woman at the top of her field, clearly enjoying her life as a financial consultant. She loved what she did—and was good at it. She charged a lot for her services, but she was worth it.

Today, Jackie looked frazzled. While aging isn't always kind, Jackie had clearly deteriorated more rapidly and profoundly than was normal for her age and for her general vitality. Her energy had waned, her hair had begun falling out, her body had expanded, and her humor had disappeared. She looked and acted beaten down by life.

With simple self-testing, the right nutritional support, and a few easily implemented interventions, Jackie was renewed before our eyes. Within a few months' time, Jackie was her old self—mature yet lovely—and we were again heartened by our mission to assist every person—preteen or octogenarian—in knowing how to make the simple adjustments that can allow them to "come back to life."

Is this you? Once, you felt young, vital, and eager to live fully. Ideas flowed, love blossomed, and the world was right. While per-

---

*All patient names are fictitious.

haps not perfect, these early years were blessed with an inner vitality, an ability to restore. You were optimistic, hopeful, and readily bounced back from the bumps of daily life.

Later, things changed. You began to feel less whole, not quite right, lost in a haze, a mere shadow of your former self.

Are you one of the millions who feel fat, fuzzy, or frazzled? Evidence is mounting that a spiraling epidemic is catching tens of millions in its escalating whirl. It drains our life force and then dumps us unceremoniously into doctors' offices. If our lab tests show normal, we may be blamed for not eating right, not thinking right, not getting enough exercise. We are given pills that obscure the real problem, leaving us vainly searching for our former fuller lives.

Fatigue, depression, weight gain, high cholesterol, low sex function, insomnia, anxiety, attention deficit, and severe menopause are common health challenges today. *Yet generally, they are not the true culprit.* What often lies at the heart of these various diagnoses, and their hundreds of related symptoms, is one underlying common cause: metabolic gland imbalance. This is what we are calling "hormone havoc."

Experts concur that one in ten Americans has some degree of endocrine gland disruption, where the various glands that are supposed to work together in harmony (such as thyroid, adrenals, and sex glands) become depleted or confused, altering their hormonal output, wreaking havoc on our lives. In our modern industrialized society, the factors contributing to this epidemic are multiple. The result is chaos. Endocrine disruption is affecting the large majority of the world population—and not only people, but animals, as well.

This situation is so daunting and so pervasive that it is increasingly missed by the medical community and by governmental agencies created to protect us. As Walt Kelly's famous comic strip character Pogo once said, "There is no problem so huge, so widespread, and so difficult to solve, that it cannot be run away from."

We are here to share some good news. As a committed doctor–nurse team, we know that endocrine gland disruption can be fixed! And as two people, like you, who have this condition (as do all three of our children), we know how much better you can feel, and how rapidly this improvement can occur.

This unique book was written to share knowledge we've gained over decades of research and personal experience—coupled with professional practice—in an easy and stepwise program. It offers an integrative hormone-balancing program with proven successful interventions for combining thyroid, adrenal, or sex hormone replacement with natural therapies. This book will help you to understand your condition, to combine simple home evaluation methods with standard medical testing for a more accurate diagnosis, and to create a plan that will enable you to move at your own pace back into your former healthy life. (For your added convenience in ordering tests or vitamins, please see pages 251 and 257 of the Appendices at the back of the book.)

If you're looking for answers, read on. This hormone-balancing program can help you take action quickly, to reclaim your youthful vigor with a new zest for facing these health challenges. Best of all, this book provides a road map to overcome them. It will help you to take a proactive role in partnership with your health providers and, ultimately, to live your best and fullest life.

A SIMPLE, OBVIOUS, AND ELEGANT SOLUTION: REBALANCE AND RECHARGE ENERGY GLANDS

To control your hormones is to control your life.
—Barry Sears, PhD, *The Zone Diet*

The dance among the endocrine hormones can seem as mysterious as the stars twinkling in their galaxies. Our mission and yours—should you choose to accept it—is to go where few doctors have dared to tread.

We wish to simplify this complexity, to help you find a new mastery over your metabolism, and thus improve the quality of your daily life. Our goal is to make this crucial topic as simple as *one, two, three.*

Here is the best news: This book can reverse *years* of unnecessary suffering and prevent even more hardship to come. The information shared is simple, safe, and effective. It is offered by experienced, caring health providers who are committed to supporting you in commanding better health care and achieving optimal health.

Recent studies have confirmed that disrupted metabolism affects at least 10 percent of our general population and up to 25 percent of menopausal women, causing them—and perhaps you—to feel tired, listless, unmotivated, overwhelmed, out of control, spacey, and fearful. Sadly, the most people suffering with metabolic imbalance remain undiagnosed, while it slowly drains their daily joy, eroding their overall quality of life. Epidemiologists also point to significant death and disease from this silent yet deadly situation if the imbalance is left untreated or is treated suboptimally.

To compound this jeopardy, many of these same metabolism-impaired people are dealing with heart disease, diabetes, arthritis, infertility, or severe menopause—commonly caused by the imbalance! Often, neither patients nor their doctors realize that beneath these more severe diagnoses lurks an easily treated hormonal problem that could be making everything else worse.

In writing this, we are speaking *not only* to the millions of people *who already have been diagnosed* with an adrenal, thyroid, or sex-hormone issue, but also to the tens of millions more who simply feel lousy and don't know why. It is our goal to demonstrate that *rebalancing your gland system can be of enormous benefit*, for dozens of debilitating everyday symptoms—many of which are currently being treated one symptom at a time (if at all) rather than being viewed as constituting a syndrome. Best of all, we aim to demonstrate that correcting this imbalance is easy, effective, and cost saving.

We know from both personal and professional experience that getting back to health can be a lifelong and sometimes frustrating journey. We wish to honor the tremendous health burden of those who have been suffering for years. We know that doctors, in their haste, often dismiss patients with multiple, seemingly unrelated symptoms, saying to them, "It's all in your head." Such a comment can affect your feelings, causing dissonance, depression, or despair.

After years of discomfort, it may be hard for you to imagine the profound and sometimes spontaneous relief that can occur through gentle rebalancing steps. Our stories, taken from actual patient experiences (names and identifying characteristics have been changed), speak volumes more eloquently than we possibly could.

With this program, you will see why the best healing occurs when all glands are properly balanced within each system—as well as in relation to each other. Then, and only then, can the endocrine system function like an orchestra, playing the various sections off one another, eventually inspiring every cell, and all aspects of our lives—physically, emotionally, mentally, spiritually.

Our self-evaluations will allow you to determine whether your thyroid, adrenal, or reproductive systems appear to be functioning at normal, subnormal, or above-normal levels. This evaluation process helps you to better comprehend your own personal metabolic profile, which is as unique as your fingerprints. You can then apply early natural interventions that offer needed relief, often without resorting to medications that can cloud the true picture and possibly cause harm.

We intend to help you become an armchair expert on cutting-edge developments, including the newest and simplified home-based saliva, blood spot, and urine testing, so you can more accurately define *your own* personal endocrine profile. Armed with this knowledge, you will be able to speak confidently to your professional health team, to command the best possible care.

These early steps, the jump start for our longer-term program, can help you feel surprisingly better within days. As an added bonus, these same steps can be repeated again and again in the future, as part of your ongoing evaluation process. If you are sufficiently improved on these first natural or over-the-counter items, then no further evaluation or treatment may be necessary at this time. Many people feel better quickly with this plan.

If, however, you do not feel adequately improved, you can then schedule time with your doctor, requesting specific blood tests that will help you to pinpoint the culprit efficiently. Based on the results, you may then advocate for a trial of prescription medicine for thyroid, reproductive, or adrenal-balancing hormones.

For those of you interested in working proactively with professionals, you will be given detailed tips on the most cost-effective and revealing blood tests, which ones to perform first, and how to interpret them optimally for improved treatment results. This step-by-step plan is focused to help you choose the tests that will provide the most essential information, giving you quicker peace of mind and saving you money.

You will be encouraged to seek out practitioners who are willing to listen closely, who will support you respectfully in your journey toward ideal endocrine balance. You will be given information on a wealth of subjects, from advocacy to xenoestrogens, interwoven into the personal stories of others with similar issues, patients who have used this program successfully. You will be encouraged to ask the right questions to command better health care. You will have the opportunity to learn, based on our decades of work with patients just like yourself, to solve the problems of feeling fat, fuzzy, or frazzled, and to feel well again—for good.

In addition, this book is intended to encourage you, as a health consumer, to find your own voice, to advocate most effectively for yourself and loved ones. It further seeks to inspire millions of health professionals to return to their roots, reclaiming the lost art of healing so desperately absent from today's health-care system.

Feeling Fat, Fuzzy, or Frazzled? is the right medicine for our fast-paced, ailing society. This powerful new program addresses the root cause of some of our most common and life-altering symptoms. It has the potential to change a great many lives—yours especially—immediately and forever. Let's start feeling better today.

AUTHOR'S APPEAL TO MEDICAL DOCTORS

Dear Colleague:

I don't know about you, but for me the practice of medicine has become much more hectic and complex than I'd like. There seems to be a constant shortage of time, but certainly no shortage of new regulations and practice constraints.

Our patients appear to be experiencing acute frustration, as well. While they are awash in increasing amounts of health information from the media and Internet, the majority of the people I see in my office feel more powerless and out of control than ever. In addition to the major illnesses, it is as if there is an epidemic of fatigue, depression, overweight, general anxiety, and decreased ability to cope with the growing demands of daily life.

Could some of this increased distress be caused by mild, hard-to-diagnose hormonal imbalances? We certainly see a large segment of the population struggling with what should be a more normal menopause. Infertility has definitely shown a dramatic increase in recent years. In my general practice, predominant complaints can be traced to depression and anxiety, often secondary to thyroid and adrenal dysfunction.

Many consumers are expressing dissatisfaction with the standard medical approach to these concerns. Couldn't we, as a profession, be more responsive to the issues that limit their enjoyment and successful pursuit of daily life? What if many of these problems are actually *symptoms* of a hormonal imbalance that we physicians could successfully treat if we were better able to diagnose it?

I've had some measure of success in recent years by listening closely to what my patients are telling me, believing what they report, and consenting to address what could be mild hormonal imbalance of thyroid gland, adrenals, or gonads. I am finding it less than useful to simply order a blood test and, based on that, tell someone "I'm sorry, your test is normal, you don't have any imbalance" when my best clinical judgment shows that they are an endocrine disaster.

The standard prescriptions for addressing these problems are often too strong, and lately I have gotten into the habit of using simple mild interventions as a first step. I've also searched for more sensitive tests than the local labs provide, and have found promising results using saliva testing for the free fraction of the hormones in question.

The first tenet of our profession is to do no harm. I believe we should attempt to help people with these simple life intrusions, despite the fact that they may not yet, if ever, be recognized as having serious named diseases. I believe it is less harmful to treat gently at the stage of early symptoms, rather than ignore the issue until the patients have lived twenty more years as "half a person."

I was amazed to discover a wide and compelling literature on the veracity of some of this new testing, and to witness the success of these mild interventions in my own practice. Occasionally these maneuvers result in the diagnosis of a severe abnormality that had not yet been tested for. Most often, however, this is not the case.

Instead, the mild alteration of thyroid, adrenal, and other hormone levels has been very helpful in allowing compromised people to feel better. At the very least, the patients feel listened to and heard, resulting in greater involvement in their own health care, and more receptivity to our long-term recommendations for healthier habits.

Just as often, however, there is an almost unexpected improvement in their general overall functioning. A person who is relieved of the hormonal cause for her anxiety is now sleeping better, getting more exercise, maybe smoking and drinking less. A person who is less hormonally depressed feels better, allowing her to now care for her ailing husband or her young children.

TO GENERAL DOCTORS

This new phase of my practice has also led to greater professional satisfaction. Subtle endocrine balance is not something the endocrinologists generally have time for. The widening epidemic of adult and childhood diabetes has burdened their practices with very sick people who need detailed and multiple interventions. Thus it might be quite appropriate for primary providers to get more involved in endocrinology as an integral part of comprehensive care. While some hormonal symptoms may seem minor to us, they could often be crucial to our patients!

TO ENDOCRINOLOGISTS

Let me say as a general practitioner that I believe many GPs would welcome more collaboration with endocrinologists in working with this particular group of patients. In confronting these complex hormonal interactions and their effects on other aspects of metabolism, I am seeing what appears to be the result of environmental xeno-estrogen and thyrotoxic synthetic chemicals. I hear from my patients that they would very much appreciate having more of your open-minded attention to what they experience as major discomforts. For some, living a decent life with energy and focus for their work and families is as important to them as proper blood sugar is for one of your diabetics.

Also, many of your diabetic patients might have occult thyroid, adrenal, and gonadal deficiencies that, when addressed more aggressively, could improve the course of their diabetic involvement. In addition to the diabetes epidemic, there is also a serious epidemic of hypothyroidism that I feel is not being handled fully by simply giving 112 milligrams (mg) of Synthroid.

I know from many of my patients that some of your patients would likely be ever so grateful if you would try harder to hear their real-life concerns. Some endocrinologists would restore greater confidence to the endocrine specialty as a whole if they would stop raising eyebrows when their patients bring these issues up for discussion. It is possible that another subspecialty is needed, so some can be "diabetologists," while others treat "minimal" gland dysfunction that feels anything but minimal to the patients experiencing them. Those patients who feel diminished by subtle glandular dysfunction and milder concerns could then work with practitioners who provide "preventive endocrinology."

You are the repositories of this key information so desperately needed by your medical colleagues and by a large segment of the population. I ask you to reach into your hearts and find some supportive time to help with this sad omission in modern medicine. It might possibly make your job easier, allowing each endocrinologist to focus on what he or she most enjoys.

FOR ALL DOCTORS

Recently I have had some measure of success in treating what appears to me to be mild endocrine imbalance. Many patients thank me for "giving them their lives back," something I had not heard much since the early days in my training, when I spent time in the ER service. I ask only that you give this idea the benefit of the doubt, meet the patients halfway, and consider recommending and supporting simple glandular interventions that can result in dramatic improvements.

I hope you will join me in encouraging our patients' educational and self-care endeavors, to inspire the greatest possible health for all.

Sincerely,
Richard L. Shames, MD

NOTES FOR NURSES, THE CAREGIVING EXPERTS

Can you imagine the power of 2.5 million nurses joining with doctors and complementary practitioners to change the face of modern medicine as it is practiced today? That is the sea change we hope to create with this book.

As a nurse for thirty years, I am convinced that we nurses have the power to transform lives and to change our medical system—more than many of us may realize. Often, when we take time with our patients, we are the first to hear about their symptoms, their pain, their dreams. In our haste, however, we can discount complaints of discomfort, perpetuating a sick care system (instead of a health-care system) that largely ignores people with subtle "dis-ease." While a limited nursing response is perfectly justifiable given the immense pressures of our work, it is also tragic. The reality is that without heart-centered nursing care, *everyone* suffers.

What if, instead, we paid close attention to "quality of life" complaints, through attentive listening and respectful involvement? I believe we would be honoring our commitment to health promotion, preventing the eventual degradation that later shows up as deeper disease. Though admittedly such attention takes more time, it can ultimately prevent a horrible toll on our patients and on ourselves. I believe that when we rush through our workdays, neglecting to share that nurturing touch that defines our art, our contributions are devalued, leaving dissatisfaction where healing seeks to grow.

A simple change of heart and focus could make an immeasurable difference, providing you with greater job satisfaction, and your patients with greater health. You are the bridge between health consumers and their doctors. As a more active advocate, you can help to ensure effective earlier intervention, the establishment of trust, and a stronger connection that can save and improve lives, all the while enriching your work life.

Learning about and employing the easily implemented tests and natural interventions outlined in this book could make a world of difference for those metabolically imbalanced patients entrusted to your care. It can help you to better understand common pitfalls of standard medical testing, which often allow people to be misdiagnosed or treated inappropriately. We nurses are in a perfect position, by virtue of our licensure, to provide details that can help people avoid illness and improve their lives.

We can gently educate doctors who may have learned endocrinology many years ago, or those who have less interest in chronic health challenges than in life-or-death situations. Inspire them to grow and enhance their skills and knowledge, their bedside manner, and their results. This is the kind of win–win–win we seek.

Nurses can be much, much more than gatekeepers or handmaidens in a "managed care" system that seems unmanaged and uncaring. By necessity, we are guardian angels for our patients. When we nurses claim our full power for greater societal health, we can offer critical guidance and advocacy as valued members of the consumer's health team. We can choose to trade in our souls, or to expand our hearts and our roles, our voices and our knowledge, to inspire healthy change.

To start, we can simply be an ally, showing the woman complaining about depression; dry skin, hair, nails; low libido; and unbearable irritability that we *do* care and that *her concerns are valid*. Even though none of these symptoms are on the order of life or death, they are incredibly real to her, and the combination of ailments leading her to feel "less like herself" may be frightening. By truly caring for her, you affirm both your and her worth simultaneously. Restored, and hopefully with the proper interventions, she can go home to care for herself, to participate in the activities that bring her joy, and ultimately to nourish loved ones, thanks to your caring touch.

Having a chronic life-sapping condition that is ignored by doctors can feel like being carried on a wave. To a normal, healthy person, being carried on a wave can seem fun, enjoyable, and exhilarating. But for a person with extreme exhaustion or nervous irritability, the wave can be terrifying. That person feels as if she is going faster than is comfortable, she can't catch her breath—and she can't stop. The pace feels wrong to her, causing her to become unduly anxious, overwrought, and fearful that she may crash at any moment, unable to find the brakes.

That is what it feels like for people with delicate endocrine conditions trying to live a normal life and to keep up with others. Since those people don't always look different, others may not understand that they are depleted, and so expect them to perform normally. To add insult to injury, when those compromised people do find the time, money, and energy to seek out medical care, they are frequently told their concerns are all in their head, and may be given Prozac, Zoloft, or stronger medications.

Our program shares basic, integrative health information that has been neglected in the quest for greater technology. It is a call to arms, for nurses and soulful caregivers, to join with each other in behalf of our patients.

Together we can inspire a powerful shift back to the roots that sustain and nurture us all. Then, with simple modifications, we can proudly live up to the promise of nursing—as powerful caregivers who provide knowledge and support, helping people to reclaim their wellness and balance while learning to protect their most precious asset, their health.

Won't you join me in awakening health consumers to the joys of creating powerful health teams, working together to restore harmony to a world in need? May this book touch your spirit and awaken your healing power, for you and those entrusted to your care, that our lives and our world will be blessed.

Karilee Shames, RN, PhD

A HEARTFELT INVITATION
TO NATURAL HEALTH PROVIDERS

As a medical doctor and registered nurse, we are delighted to see more and more alternative health practitioners contributing to this arena of subtle hormone balancing. Your involvement, support, focus, attention, and expertise are desperately needed. Not only does this problem represent an epidemic where millions of people are suffering, but worse, millions are suffering *needlessly*, which is unconscionable. Modern medicine, as presently structured, is simply not equipped to diagnose and treat these mild hormonal imbalances.

People need better options than their physicians generally provide. They need more support than physicians give. There needs to be greater freedom of choice among a wide variety of diagnostic and therapeutic tools. Patients are hungry for this, and they are demanding it.

You have a special role in the evolving model. You can offer a variety of strategies to complement their more traditional medical care. This blending of alternative and traditional therapies has proved more powerful than either would be alone.

You are in the best possible position to work with patients' belief systems, to emphasize the importance of nutrition, emotions, exercise, and bodywork, of adding spiritual practices and finding balance in their lives. It is simply time for you to step forward and claim your proper place in the evolving model, as an integral and essential part of the consumer's health team, as wise counselors and healers, providing thoughtful insight with compassionate care.

In addition to your work with patients, and perhaps more challenging, you may also need to reach out and create a bridge to the medical doctors. Many physicians have perhaps been too busy treating life- and limb-threatening diseases to give proper attention to more subtle endocrine issues. Helpful in this endeavor is to bring up any research articles that you have had time to review, perhaps respectfully forwarding them to the more conventional practitioner who is also caring for your patient. Doctors often want to be providing evidence-based care, but don't have time to seek out the most recent evidence that you may be aware of.

In addition, your offer to help the medical doctor with an agitated patient, perhaps in need of nutritional counseling or stress reduction, may be more appreciated than you could have imagined, especially if you can find ways to comfortably collaborate. You will need to stand tall, conveying respect not only for the other practitioners, but also for the fine tradition you represent in your professional field. Ideally, we will all be considered as equal team members, including the consumer at the center of our care.

Rich, as a physician, really appreciates receiving messages that an alternative practitioner treating one of his patients has made certain suggestions, perhaps that the patient could benefit additionally from some lymphatic massage or Pilates training. In this way, we as professionals are able to coordinate and demonstrate our respect for each other, while better treating the patient and expanding knowledge.

We realize that this may feel like bowing to medical doctors, who tend to see themselves as the ultimate authority. However, this kind of bridging and diplomacy can bring rich rewards. We are hopeful there will come the time when it will become a situation of mutuality, wherein all practitioners consult with each other for the best results for the shared consumer (whom we are encouraging to be less "patient"). We urge you to step up to the plate and to become more involved in the needed revolution in health care.

It appears that today we have an enormous environmental-endocrine problem that the medical doctors are mostly not interested in or prepared to deal with. Your role in stemming the tide of this epidemic is crucial.

Please read this material carefully, and know that while you may not agree with every single statement, it is a beginning in building bridges between your field and that of physicians and other caregivers. Chiropractors would use a more hands-on approach, alleviating musculoskeletal blockages impacting nerves and energy flow. Acupuncturists would place needles appropriately, perhaps using moxa to release blockages. Bodyworkers would each approach the same patient in a unique way, depending on his or her personal training. Osteopathic and naturopathic doctors and practitioners have made wonderful contributions to this field, and have been so helpful to us in our evolution. We truly enjoy this rich collaboration. Through a multidisciplinary approach, consumers can make better informed choices.

For those practitioners who are much further along than we are in this arena of subtle hormone balance, please realize that *this book is a deliberate oversimplification*. We are attempting to engage the lay public in the realization that their hormones—and not just sex hormones—could be involved in many of the conditions for which they are now taking prescription symptom-relievers. Moreover, we are trying to get the point across that a major reason for so much hormonal imbalance may well be the increasing pollution of the air, food, and water, with synthetic chemicals that are surprisingly hormonally active. Once they're informed, we encourage consumers and providers to become politically active in behalf of our struggling planet.

We need your help, not simply as practitioners for suffering people, but also as voices of professional outrage. We intend, through this project and others, to command accountability on the part of our government and corporations, to reduce the number, quantity, and toxicity of these industrial pollutants flooding over us all. The concern for the general welfare of our nation and world *must* outweigh concerns for industry and financial gain. Thank you for doing your part in this critical time.

Karilee and Richard Shames

THE 3-LEGGED STOOL— A NEW MODEL FOR BALANCING GLANDS

Hypotheses are nets; only he who casts will catch.
—Friedrich von Hardenberg

The endocrine system consists of a dozen organs that secrete more than twenty different messenger molecules, yet there are *three* glands that have overriding importance. Working properly, these three constitute a solid foundation upon which the rest of our hormonal and metabolic health is built.

These three energy-regulating glands are the thyroid, adrenals, and sex glands (ovaries and testes). They can be viewed as a three-legged stool upon which rests our ability to feel balanced and to function effectively in our daily lives.

Ideally, the 3-legged stool provides a sturdy and level surface. If any one leg is too high, or too low, then the stool slants, and you no longer have a stable surface for what rests on top. In this case, what rests on top is the integrity and proper functioning of our entire metabolic system.

One major cause of this increase in energy hormone challenges is the constant stress of modern life. Our adrenals are the "fight or flight" glands that secrete excess cortisol under duress, flooding the system with biochemicals that affect our nervous system, resulting in increased anxiety and irritability. Depletion of the adrenal gland causes the thyroid gland to compensate, draining it, as well.

Another reason for today's hormone disruption epidemic, causing one or more legs to be unequal in length, is environmental pollution.

For example, a sensitive person whose thyroid gland is slowed due to exposure to PCBs (polychlorinated biphenyls, alarmingly pervasive in our environment today) will have a three-legged stool with the thyroid leg shorter than normal, slowing metabolism, resulting in multiple uncomfortable symptoms. The most obvious changes include the following:

- excess weight
- severe fatigue
- depression
- a sense of tiredness than can become exhaustion
- dry skin, hair, and nails, as well as a variety of skin conditions
- a host of female problems (difficult periods, bad menopause, PMS, infertility, miscarriage), and low libido in both men and women

In like manner, an adrenal-sensitive person may suffer exposure to dioxin (common in pesticides), resulting in altered adrenal hormone production, which then causes excess stress response and lesser ability to cope. This person now has a 3-legged stool with the adrenal leg shorter than the others.

A third person, like many baby-boomers, may have lived where DDT mosquito spraying was popular. Though the pesticide was banned in the United States in 1972, it remains persistent in the environment. She may now be suffering severe menopause after years of infertility and menstrual problems caused by the hormone disruptive properties of this chemical. Her sensitive reproductive glands have been under attack! She is an example of someone whose 3-legged stool has a shortened leg for sex hormones.

To simplify our program, these three individuals represent what we are calling three different *endo-types*:

"Feeling fat" thyroid-driven **Physical** endo-type
"Fuzzy-thinking" sex gland–driven **Mental** endo-type
"Fried and frazzled" adrenal-driven **Emotional** endo-type

Our goal is to simplify a complex situation: hormonal imbalance. Notice that in addition to naming a specific organ, we have added the words *physical, mental,* and *emotional.* The reason for doing this is that in addition to the major symptom (fat, fuzzy, or frazzled), we refer to the major realm of one's life that is largely impacted (physical, mental, or emotional).

Thyroid-driven endo-types frequently have largely *physical* symptoms, including weight problems, body temperature–regulation challenges, and difficulties manufacturing the physical energy to run their system. In essence, a thyroid-driven imbalance could also be called the **physical** endo-type. In this book, we have created three characters to represent these main endo-types. The **Physical** endo-type, or thyroid-challenged person, is named *Ph*oebe.

Sex gland–driven endo-types frequently have the *mental* symptoms of foggy thinking, memory loss, inability to concentrate, and difficulty with focus, resulting in challenges with the mental energy to clearly run the brain. In essence, a sex gland–driven imbalance could also be called the **Mental** endo-type, who in our stories is represented by *M*eredith.

Adrenal-driven endo-types frequently have the *emotional* symptoms of anger and irritability, or fear and anxiety, resulting in challenges with having stable emotional energy to run their lives smoothly. In essence, the adrenal-driven imbalance could also be called the **Emotional** endo-type, who in our examples is called *Em*ily.

These examples represent only the main—or pure—endo-types. While many people have one main endo-type, others have a mixture, wherein two or even three legs are out of balance. For clarity, however, we identify and describe traits of each of the three main endo-types individually, until the last chapter, where we share more about how to address multigland involvement.

Chapter 1 introduces and names the problem we are addressing.

Chapter 2 identifies the sources of this problem.

Chapter 3 presents self-evaluations to begin to get a sense of which glands might be involved and causing such disruption, allowing you to figure out your apparent endo-type.

Chapter 4 discusses recommended testing to confirm your actual endo-type.

Chapter 5 provides initial general remedies, first steps to help all endo-types begin to nourish their glands rapidly, so you can feel better fast and set the stage for ongoing success.

Chapters 6, 7, and 8 offer individual rebalancing tools to help you reclaim your full health. Chapter 6 has specific recommendations for **physical** endo-type challenges, chapter 7 for **mental** endo-types, and chapter 8 for **emotional** endo-types to reclaim and restore their health.

Chapters 9 through 11 offer long-term strategies to help you maintain your improvement forever. Chapter 9 shares long-term suggestions for **physical** endo-types, 10 for **mental** endo-types, and 11 for **emotional** endo-types.

Chapter 12 makes final recommendations for all endo-types. It summarizes the most important concepts of this program, encouraging you to maintain your wellness forever, while feeling and looking your best. For those who would like to use their newly acquired vitality toward creating a healthier world, this chapter provides inspiration and ideas.

Many times, taking care of the most urgent symptoms allows you to return to a full and comfortable life. However, if you continue to have symptoms, and you know which other gland or glands might be involved, you may elect to work on another endo-type at that phase of your healing journey, and then tackle the specific challenges of that type. Much like the peeling of an onion, eventually you will uncover the culprit and restore balance to the problem that was causing such concern.

As a useful model, consider that if *any* of the legs of this crucial 3-legged stool is too long or too short, your out-of-balance system can benefit from restorative measures. If more than one leg is out of balance, we offer a stepwise process to help you comfortably stabilize this delicate hormonal dance, symbolized by the 3-legged stool.

Working with this model, you can further improve metabolic meltdown through dietary support, stress reduction, enjoyable exercise, vitamin, mineral, and herbal supplementation, and many other exciting approaches to make this as rewarding as possible for you!

What we are providing here is news you can use. Our main goal is to bring this hormonal dance alive for you and your loved ones—physically, mentally, emotionally, and spiritually.

As integrative medical professionals, we want to see you live your fullest life possible. We are convinced that as you claim greater health, you will contribute to a healthier society. Together, we can build a more peaceful and balanced world, a treasure we will care for lovingly and leave proudly as a legacy for future generations.

INTRODUCTION TO STEP I

This program is divided into three major steps:

- Step I: The Jump Start of <u>Initial</u> Evaluations to pinpoint your problem and to help you feel better right away.
- Step II: <u>Intermediate</u> Rebalancing Tools, allowing you to not only alleviate symptoms but also to restore your glands.
- Step III: Sustaining <u>Long-Term</u> Success: Maintenance Practices to help you retain your improved health status forever.

This first step—**The Jump Start**—defines the challenge and its likely causes. To understand the cause is the key to fixing the problem. Once you have identified your specific condition, you will be given starting measures to begin correcting your imbalance immediately. These include basic nutrition, such as vitamins, minerals, and quick dietary adjustments, along with other immediate actions to set the stage for success.

There can be *hundreds of other common symptoms* related to hormonal imbalance of thyroid, adrenal, or sex glands. Even if you're not feeling fat, fuzzy, or frazzled, this first step may be surprisingly beneficial to you in revealing the hormonal connections to these other discomforting symptoms. May it give you a jump start on your return to optimal health.

Day 1: Name the Problem
Day 2: Determine the Cause
Day 3: Estimate Your Endo-Type Using Self-Evaluations
Day 4: Confirm Your Endo-Type with Simple Home Tests
Day 5: Set the Stage for Success

STEP I
THE FIVE-DAY JUMP START

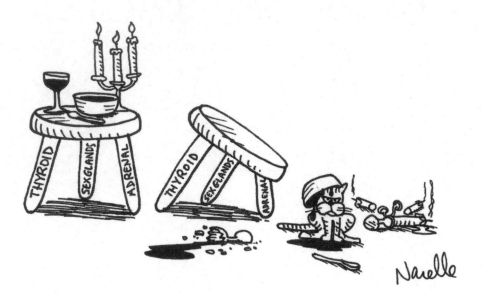

CHAPTER 1

DAY 1 OF YOUR JUMP START
NAME THE PROBLEM

I balanced all, brought all to mind.

—William Butler Yeats

Three women sat in a waiting room, flipping through magazines. Suddenly Phoebe, short and round with red hair, groaned loudly, causing the others to look up. "I don't believe it," she said. "It's a constant barrage of simple-sounding rhetoric about how to be healthy. Now even Dr. Phil has jumped on the diet bandwagon. These experts act as if all you have to do is eat better and exercise more, and everything will be perfect! I did all of that for years, and nothing worked. Wouldn't it be great if it were just that easy? We'd all be perfect!"

Meredith, a thin, weary-looking brunette sitting across from her, chuckled. "I hear you. Weight wasn't my problem, but I've been frustrated, too. I was doing pretty well until the last few years. Suddenly the mom who could juggle everything couldn't even remember to pick up her son, who's waiting in the dark at the baseball field. My thinking got so foggy, the kids teased me, saying I had early Alzheimer's! Nothing helped."

The third woman, Emily, listened quietly. Young, dark-haired, and attractive, she nodded in agreement. "I'm not having memory loss, and weight's never been my big issue either. But lately things have been pretty aggravating! I'm only twenty-nine, and I've been feeling more frazzled than my mom ever was, even after she had three babies! I used to be so upbeat; then I started to snap at anyone who dared to cross my path. I became a nervous wreck most the time, and I hated it, but couldn't seem to do anything about it. I tried over-the-counter re-laxants during the day and even some sleeping pills at night. It just didn't work! With all those changes, I felt like I was losing my mind! It's only recently that I'm starting to feel human again, thanks to this endo-type balancing."

As they introduced themselves, the women realized that while they each experienced very different symptoms, they all had a few things in common. Each had visited doctor after doctor, seeking relief, to no avail. Worse yet, these ongoing difficulties were affecting their social and work lives on a daily basis.

Each woman, after coming to our clinic, had uncovered an underly-ing metabolic challenge that was causing her seemingly untreatable problems. Fortunately, each was now beginning to reclaim her health, functioning and feeling better more of the time, with renewed confi-dence in her future.

The older women, Phoebe and Meredith, had spent years trying to cope with their respective health challenges. Emily had only recently be-come symptomatic. All had felt overwhelmed and unable to perform where previously they had excelled. They had secretly experienced a sense of demoralization and fear, wondering if recovery would ever be possible and, if not, what would become of their lives.

EXCESS WEIGHT: THE "FAT" (PHYSICAL) CHALLENGE

For Phoebe, the culprit was excess weight, with its concomitant lack of energy and libido. Since puberty, she had been teased for her short round figure. Her face was now puffy, adding to the image of someone a bit too plump. She had attended nutrition classes for years, and was seeing a counselor to deal with the emotional aspects of her situation, including the hurt she felt in response to her husband's disparaging remarks about her expanding body. Nonetheless, she found that she was becoming even larger, which clearly had a negative impact on her self-esteem.

In reality, few health challenges are as demoralizing and upsetting to people as persistent weight problems, particularly in our thin-worshipping society. Compared with other health concerns, obesity ranks foremost in frequency for various reasons. As a society, our high-fat, low-nutrient diets eaten on the run, coupled with larger portion sizes, add to our weight. In addition, the accelerating pace of life makes it exceptionally difficult to find time to exercise adequately. Moreover, as will be further explained in chapter 2, many artificial hormonelike substances in our environment directly interfere with proper metabolism.

Americans today are the among the most overweight people on the planet, plagued with a variety of related health epidemics, including those of heart disease, diabetes, and high blood pressure. If you are overweight, you may want to consider the possibility that a metabolic imbalance is causing you those extra pounds. If the cause for your overweight is glandular, proper hormone balancing makes it much more likely that you will live longer, more healthfully, and will enjoy life more fully.

Commonly, what is attributed to genetics, personality, or habit can actually be *glandular* in origin.

The likelihood of having off-balance glands is increasingly worthy of our focused attention. Recent statistics show that 10 to 12 percent of our U.S. population (28 to 35 million people) suffer from some form of metabolic malfunction.

Phoebe had been overweight almost her entire life despite countless diets and weight loss programs. In her teen years, counselors suspected compulsive overeating, but that was never the case. She was simply heavy and couldn't lose a pound, no matter how little she ate or how much she exercised. Now, in her midlife, she also had to deal with irregular periods.

In fact, only recently had she discovered our clinic, where she began to receive treatment for low metabolism, despite "normal" tests. Trained as a nurse, Phoebe—like many health professionals—had an unrealistic faith in the absolute accuracy of blood tests.

As you will see, her new willingness and insight to look beyond test results have made all the difference in her life. After working with the thyroid balancing tools presented in this book, her menstrual discomfort mellowed dramatically. Within a year, she had lost forty-three pounds and felt great.

What pleased her most was keeping the weight off and feeling better than she had felt in years. Not only is she now enjoying her new shape, but she also likes being able to exercise more, feeling lighter, energetic, and more comfortable in her body. Needless to say, her relationship has also improved. Now, she is able to actually tease her husband about his *paunchy waist.*

Phoebe is an example of what we refer to as the thyroid hormone endocrine profile, or simply the **physical** endo-type. Often people in this category experience a wide variety of symptoms, including fatigue; overweight; depression; dry skin, hair, and nails; as well as an intense sense of malaise, especially around puberty, menopause, or during other life changes. The majority of people in this category experience weight gain, despite normal eating habits and reasonable exercise. When the thyroid slows, so do you.

The thyroid is a walnut-size butterfly-shaped gland at the base of the throat. It functions as the "gas pedal" for the whole body by secreting energy hormones that control the speed of every metabolic process in every cell and every organ.

While a glandular imbalance was clearly part of Phoebe's excess weight, could it also have something to do with Meredith's foggy thinking? Is it possible that Emily's recent inability to cope might also have a glandular component? Let's consider their stories.

LOSING MENTAL CLARITY:
THE "FUZZY" (MENTAL) CHALLENGE

Meredith was thirty-nine years old, a single mom with two young teens. She had been very involved in their schooling, often volunteering on various committees. In fact, Meredith was frequently the mom who organized soccer outings, never missed a game, yet also was able to work into the night, concentrating on the kids' homework in a clear and organized manner. Recently, however, she was finding that she could not keep up with the everyday demands of life in her usual methodical and focused way.

Meredith's previous adaptations to parenting were no longer fully effective. There was now just too much to do, and too little ability to think things over as carefully as she had done in the past. In fact, Meredith began to have major memory difficulties. She would neglect to bring the grocery list to the store. She would forget her plans to meet with friends downtown, and on one occasion, left her son waiting alone at the baseball field past dark.

Not incidentally, all of this began when her periods became somewhat irregular and heavy. Her gynecologist had called it a mild case of dysfunctional uterine bleeding, and had put her on birth control pills to regulate her cycle. This, however, made her feel worse. Now she experienced increased water retention and her usually lumpy breasts became uncomfortably swollen and tender, both symptoms of estrogen excess. Her sleep was more irregular, as well.

Meredith represents what we call the sex-hormone endocrine profile, or simply the **mental** endo-type. This is where a person loses "spark," often finding it difficult to think clearly or stay focused. Commonly, it is a low level of estrogen or testosterone that affects memory. High levels, however, can also hurt mental function in unusually sensitive people like Meredith.

Despite having more regular periods after taking the birth control pills, Meredith's extra estrogen led to a further cognitive decline. She began to leave food burning on the stove, and could no longer follow conversations easily or balance her checkbook. She would enter a room and not remember why she had decided to come in there. She felt "foggy" in her thinking, spacey and disconnected.

Fortunately, after coming to our clinic, she began to understand that her hormones were causing much of this fogginess. Her brain was exquisitely sensitive to estrogen levels, which were already excessive before going onto the birth control pills. Taking them resulted in more estrogen, and therefore increased memory loss.

As will become apparent in following chapters, small interventions in nutrition—balanced later with some herbal medicines and natural progesterone cream—allowed her to return to a more normal existence, focused in her daily life, and increasingly able to handle her daily demands.

The reproductive glands are housed in the lower abdomen, where they secrete hormones that provide focus and stamina for social interactions and reproduction. These hormones can include estrogen, testosterone, and progesterone, all of which exist in both sexes.

Other typical symptoms of female sex-gland imbalances can include irregular or painful periods, fertility challenges, difficult transitions such as puberty, childbirth, and menopause. For men, sex-gland challenges often manifest as a loss of vitality, low stamina, and perhaps a disconnection with one's sense of purpose. Both sexes frequently experience lowered libido, as well.

FEELING STRESSED: THE "FRAZZLED" (EMOTIONAL) CHALLENGE

Emily, age twenty-nine, was actively involved in an exciting and demanding career as a stockbroker. Unmarried and dating, she kept herself constantly busy, taking business classes at her local community college, in addition to a stretching class twice a week. Her life suddenly became difficult when she was transferred from Denver to San Fran-

cisco, and was asked to take on a supervisory role. Though her promotion was welcome, she found the additional stress overwhelming.

Once at her San Francisco location, she started to have difficulty coping with the inevitable challenges of a move, including adapting to a faster-paced environment. The unpacking, constant search for things that were hard to find, and disarray caused her to become progressively unglued. Her new role at work involved making very difficult managerial decisions, with little support from supervisors at a time of a downturn in the market. Key employees were upset, some leaving, others clearly disgruntled and antagonistic. Several were blatantly taking out their frustrations on her.

Her usual pleasant demeanor became aggressive and intolerant. She would easily erupt in bursts of anger. Little things set her off. She developed frequent upset stomach and headaches. She felt totally stressed and further frustrated from having a medical problem that doctors couldn't do much about. They told her all her tests were normal. They gave her strong acid blockers for GERD (gastrointestinal reflux disease), which wasn't very helpful. She had shoulder and neck pain, with recurrent headaches and difficulty sleeping. Neurologists found nothing wrong, and they advised her to take tranquilizers and Advil, which not only didn't help, but also made her stomach worse.

Emily was at her wit's end. She felt hostile and agitated. Friends were amazed at how different she had become.

Emily is an example of the adrenal hormone endocrine profile or what we call the **emotional** endo-type.

The adrenals are two grape-size glands that sit at the top of each kidney. Their function is to provide the messenger molecules for coping with stress. Their secretions control what is known as the "fight or flight" response, as well as carbohydrate metabolism, fluid balance, and immune function.

As it turns out, everything from glucose and fat storage to kidney function are affected by the adrenal flow. Excess adrenal can make people very jittery. Too little adrenal can make a person unable to handle any stress or confrontation. Disruption of this critical balance causes a great deal of what we know as anxiety, fear, and rage.

THE DANCE OF THE HORMONES

Endocrine balance is crucial to the proper functioning of our immune system. In fact, the integration and organization of our unique and amazingly complex selves are under direct control of the endocrine glands. They unify the other systems by coordinating functions among the various organs and body parts.

While all these glands take their orders from, and communicate with, the brain, it is actually through the guidance of our hormones that the brain functions. Ultimately, these chemical messengers direct brain activity, impacting the development of traits that shape us as individuals. This hormonal interplay can determine whether we live a very full vibrant life or become a shadow of our potential self.

All animals can be irrevocably affected if assaulted by the wrong hormones at critical times. Mammals in utero are exquisitely sensitive to minute shifts in hormone levels. In considering our three main "energy hormones" (adrenal, thyroid, sex), any one of them can be deficient, wrongly underproducing or overproducing in relation to the other two. This lack of balance commonly results in feeling fat, fuzzy, or frazzled.

In addition to the separate actions of each of these above hormones, there is another overriding factor that must be considered. *If the thyroid is low, the adrenal and sex hormones can also be low as result.* This is one of the side effects of low thyroid, since the thyroid gland fuels the actions of the other two. This simple yet profound fact is very commonly overlooked in medical consultations.

Hormones constantly interact with each other to help maintain balance. If your adrenal is low, although you may have enough thyroid hormone, the thyroid won't act properly. Thyroid needs a normal amount of adrenal hormone to be converted from its transport state (T4) to its purely active state (T3).

Furthermore, considering sex hormones, thyroid function can be diminished if your estrogen is too high. Estrogen dominance increases thyroid-binding proteins in the blood. This results in having less thyroid hormone available to the cells and tissues.

How Common Are These Problems?

According to researchers at the Columbia Presbyterian Medical Center in New York, one in ten Americans—more than 28 million people—are known to have struggles with gland imbalance. Yet experts tell us that in any given population, *half* the people with this condition remain undiagnosed. It is sometimes called a "hidden epidemic."

This means that it is quite likely that almost 50 million Americans are at risk. If you are reading this book, then you or someone you love or work with is no doubt affected.

Previous medical studies have reported that approximately one in every four menopausal women had some noticeable degree of thyroid imbalance, a definite contributor to the cause of obesity. Glandular difficulties, similar to other chronic health problems, become more severe and more common with age. It is virtually impossible to estimate the number of people impacted by this slowdown or disruption of these three main glands, but there is a growing understanding that many in the geriatric population can be greatly helped by some gentle hormonal rebalancing.

The young, however, are not exempt. Increased weight and terrible acne are classic symptoms of hormone imbalance. They also are typical of young people going through puberty. Fertility problems affecting men and women in their childbearing years are rapidly, heartbreakingly, and dramatically on the rise. In addition, many postpartum depressions are actually postpartum thyroid abnormalities.

Additionally, the astounding surge in incidence of childhood diabetes, autism, and ADD-related conditions speaks to the sensitivity of the younger segment of our population. It is now estimated that one of every three people in the U.S. population is obese; one in four complains of anxiety-related problems. Again these are both cardinal symptoms of gland disturbance.

The Medical Response to a Mushrooming Epidemic

Having spent years working with people in pain, we firmly believe that there are better solutions to many current health problems than are being provided by the standard Western medical model. Millions of health consumers are receiving substandard care, even from well-intentioned, seasoned practitioners. To protect yourself, you must better understand your own health needs.

Every day for decades, we have seen women and men trudge into our office filled with anguish and despair. They have been through the mill, seeing doctor after doctor with poor results. Some actually feel worse after taking medicines directed merely toward symptom relief, without attention to the underlying cause of the problem. If you search beyond the obvious to determine this underlying cause, in one of every ten people you will find some measure of gland imbalance.

We hope you will use this book to arm yourself with remedies and techniques that do not always require a physician or prescription to help you feel better. In fact, you could be one of the many people who experience rapid improvement after adding just a few crucial nutrients or adjustments to your daily program.

Standard tests are not always able to diagnose mild metabolic glandular imbalance. The 3-legged integrative model, not generally taught to physicians, often provides more lasting benefits.

Modern Medicine Missing the Boat

In addition to modern medicine missing the hormonal connection to many illnesses, there is too often a denial of the potential dangers of harsh pharmaceuticals so lightly provided to patients. Doctors generally have not been adequately trained to consider the relationship among past chemical exposures, personal history, familial patterns, or subtle allergic sensitivities. Unfortunately, the blame for causing the condition is all too often wrongly placed on the patient. In a sense, patients and providers alike have become victims of a myopic system.

One of the main difficulties is that our present medical system professes to have neither the time nor the money to conduct a sufficiently comprehensive evaluation of a patient, despite the fact that the right testing could uncover the root cause of a person's lifelong suffering, saving both the patient and the system years of aggravation and expense. Another is that modern medicine has generally focused on high-tech solutions and the most severe medical conditions, largely ignoring milder, harder-to-diagnose difficulties that "simply" compromise quality of life. The standard range of normal just does not apply to every person equally. The result is that regular blood tests frequently miss the problem. That's right! Your tests *may show normal*, but your symptoms may be pointing you toward the truth.

With the current wide "normal" ranges for hormone blood tests, the assumption seems to be that every person has the same genetic potential, inherited possibility, and life experience. In reality, nothing could be further from the truth.

While we can't see emotions, or the biochemicals that cause them, we know they exist, and we can see their effects in our behaviors. Similarly while we cannot see the hormones flowing in our bloodstream, we can see their "footprints" in certain health patterns.

You cannot count on your doctor to bring up the possibility of thyroid, adrenal, or sex hormonal imbalance as a likely culprit in your feeling fat, fuzzy, or frazzled. Most physicians have never been appropriately trained to do so. Similarly, most doctors are less than fully informed about the newer diagnostic tests, or the milder yet often more effective vitamin, mineral, or herbal interventions for restoring proper function.

In reality, a great many physicians are held captive, in a certain sense, to highly conservative and standardized training, rendering them unable to practice as freely as they may prefer. Governing bodies evaluate doctors' performances based on how closely the doctor follows the "standards of practice" for various situations and locations. Therefore, it becomes virtually impossible for a health professional to inject newer approaches without raising skeptical, sometimes hostile, eyebrows in the medical community.

As a health consumer, you need to understand that it can be *very* risky for a doctor to try some newer ways of working. The challenge for practitioners who do seek to develop newer models becomes that of figuring out how to practice in an innovative and supportive manner while remaining somewhat below the radar in a financially driven system that resists change. The result is that doctors are notorious for proceeding cautiously, with good reason. We encourage you to be aware of this and to learn how to make the best of it. To this end, we provide you with ample suggestions and even some useful scripts for specific situations and interactions.

A BEGINNING SOLUTION

Should you determine that this endocrine-disruption issue is indeed part of your problem, this eye-opening journey is guaranteed to empower you, giving you the chance to take charge of your medical care, and to reclaim your precious and long-compromised health.

First Steps

As simple beginning steps, *we recommend that you start keeping daily records* of what is going on regarding the way you look, feel, act, and think. You might get a notebook just for the purpose of documenting your journey to health. In it, include thoughts, dreams, conversations, confrontations, and any information that may prove relevant to your case.

- Create a list of any symptoms you are presently experiencing.
- Next, discuss changes you perceive in yourself, whether they be physical, mental, or emotional. (You can make a column for each of these categories.)
- Then, describe your attempts to ameliorate these problems, using medical protocols, alternative therapies, natural remedies, imagery, movement, or whatever else you have tried.

Next, *begin to organize your medical records.*

- Contact all the offices in which you have been a patient, and request copies of any reports or doctors' notes revealing the problems relating to possible gland involvement.
- Ask them to send actual test scores, not simply notes or a letter about these tests.
- Add to this information any previous exposures you've had to

chemicals, early childhood illnesses, or previous diagnoses you've received.

Document unusual challenges you may have experienced with puberty, childbirth, menstruation, or menopause. Describe any sexual concerns or PMS difficulties.

Now, begin to *seek information from family members*.

- Who has had diabetes or thyroid problems?
- Has anyone been diagnosed with an autoimmune disease, such as lupus, multiple sclerosis, rheumatoid arthritis, migraine headaches, ulcerative colitis, or Crohn's disease?
- Has there been severe childbirth or other female problems, fertility or menstrual/menopausal problems in female family members?
- Are there any cases of premature gray hair (before age forty)? Early graying, mitral valve problems, or carpal tunnel often indicate a familial pattern of gland imbalance.
- Ascertain if there has been cretinism (baby born of low-thyroid mother, with resultant mental deficits and physical syndrome), Addison's (adrenal gland disease often with immune causation), or other serious gland concerns.
- Become aware of familial patterns of behavior, diet, thought, and other manifestations, such as mental illness, that could signal metabolic issues.

To better understand your individual situation, we now discuss our glands and how they work. We will explore the mutuality that exists between metabolic challenges and our emotions, rounding out a discussion of the important interconnections and showing ultimately how you can conquer feeling fat, fuzzy, or frazzled.

HOW YOUR GLANDS SHOULD WORK

Messenger molecules make us who we are. The wrong messages make us sleepy, lethargic, spacey, easily overwhelmed, or any combination of these.

In her book *Molecules of Emotion*, Candace Pert, PhD, tells of her amazing journey as a researcher at the National Institutes of Health. As a graduate student, she laid the foundation for the discovery of endorphins, the body's own painkillers and ecstasy-inducing chemicals.

Authoritative and irreverent, she was amazed that lay people came in droves to her seminars and lectures, wanting desperately to be more in charge of their health, deeply disappointed in the failures of modern medicine to deliver on many of its promises. Her work beautifully weaves together the mental and the physical, two seemingly disparate schools of thought. Their separation is often referred to as Cartesian dualism or mind–body split.

One overpowering old belief is that illness is created in the body and needs to be addressed physically. With the rise of modern psychology, a contrasting view asserts a mental origin for many health concerns, believing that in order to fix illness in the body, one must start with the mind.

From a physical scientist's viewpoint, Dr. Pert shares the magnificence of atoms, molecules, and chemical bonds. Her perspective honors the mysterious nature of our biochemicals, addressing emotions, and explaining their intricate connection to chemicals in continuous flow between the body and brain. She brings together body and mind, heart and spirit, supporting the view of human beings as whole, complex, and multidimensional.

These concepts help us to understand how critical it is that each person finds his biochemical balance, restoring health and harmony, in order to live a life with meaning and purpose. *Hormone* is derived from the Greek word meaning "to urge on." In this sense, the chemical messenger made in one part of the body travels to another, carrying an important message, urging various organs and glands to make biochemical adjustments.

These messages are part of the body's internal conversation, encouraging trillions of cells to work together in some degree of harmony rather than chaos. And when the wrong messages are sent, there can be devastating results.

**Our glandular output largely defines who
we are. It affects our emotions, mental clarity,
physical abilities, and even how we look.**

Some folks might feel depressed, irritable, or highly anxious. Others may suffer at the mercy of reproductive hormones, which can be responsible for sexually aggressive behaviors or amazingly dramatic mood swings. All these symptoms, and many more, can result from an excess or deficiency of one hormone, *or* from an out-of-balance hormonal triad.

The Triad Model: Keys, Locks, and Molecular Magic

While we have many hormones in our body, this book focuses on three major endocrine hormones, the secretions from the adrenal, thyroid, and reproductive glands. These three glands are regulated by the brain via relay through the pituitary, at the base of the brain.

This gland trio is absolutely essential for the function of everything else in the body. The *thyroid* is responsible for body temperature, growth, and the speed of chemical reactions. The *adrenals* control how a person interfaces with any physical or psychological stress. The *sex-gland hormones* regulate much more than reproduction. They are responsible for clarity and focus of brain tissue, strength and stability of muscles, and the quality and joy of our lives.

Recall that one purpose of these endocrine glands is to enable the brain to effectively regulate messenger activities at distant sites. The brain is constantly monitoring the blood to assure appropriate levels of messenger molecules. When it senses a need for more of one particular type of molecule, the brain signals the pituitary to stimulate hormone production in the specific distant gland that makes the necessary substance. In this way, the producing gland, whether thyroid, adrenal, or sex gland, secretes more of the needed chemical, thereby maintaining an exquisite balance in the system.

The molecules released from our endocrine glands communicate back and forth constantly between the brain, nervous system, and sensitive tissues of our body. They are what we will be calling chemical messengers. They can provide the spark of life or, in some instances, the kiss of death.

**There are hundreds of messenger molecules
made in various parts of the body. Each functions
as a key that will open one particular lock.**

Adrenaline is an example of a messenger molecule, with a simple one-ring molecular structure. Slightly more complex would be two rings attached together with three or four atoms of iodine; this is called thyroid hormone. Even more complex, yet still considered a simple molecule, is the four-ring structure of estrogen or testosterone. A very complex molecule, with many amino acids strung into an extremely long chain, folded in a complicated manner, is the messenger molecule insulin, responsible for allowing sugar to enter our cells, providing energy for life.

While the above messenger molecules are the keys, the lock is the hormone receptor, located either on the cell surface or inside the cell. Its job, once unlocked, is to signal certain cell machinery into action. For this to happen, the precise key must enter its corresponding lock. When the hormone key unlocks its specific receptor, the result is some change in cell activity.

Thus, receptor sites on cells function like sensor stations, where chemical messengers have their effects. This occurs when messenger molecules attach to a receptor site, creating a disturbance, which "tickles" the receptor into rearranging itself, changing its shape until the information enters into the cell. This lock-and-key process is known as binding, which Pert playfully refers to as "molecular sex."

Sometimes the new action is quite profound, as when messenger molecules release the reading of the DNA genetic code.

**When the messenger molecules bind on their receptor
sites, the result is that the information contained within
that particular cell's chromosomes is now causing the
expression of that person's genetic potential.**

How we think, how we live, how we move—all of these are driven by a subtle force that ancient cultures referred to as the "life force," the "thousand-year-old healer within." It is the power to sustain us and keep us whole.

All our activities, from creating masterpiece paintings to heart-wrenching poetry, from drafting magnificent buildings to birthing beautiful children, derive from the life force sparked by our inner creativity. From politics to lovemaking, all the energy for life is inspired by this hormonal dance.

Within the DNA are encoded ancient memories of our familial history, the record of human evolution, and our unique genetic combination. It defines who we are, at our highest moment, and what we are capable of becoming. The expression of all this genetic material is dependent upon the binding of particular hormones at given sites, activating the reading, and therefore the expression, of each human's uniqueness and possibilities. Our brains, our glands, our heart—all the muscles, bones, joints, and connections are dependent upon receiving the right amount of hormone at the right time.

If you have been feeling less than whole, it could be because something as basic as your brain function has been slowed by hormonal imbalance. Correcting this mental sluggishness with appropriate hormonal balancing can restore you to your previous healthy self.

How These Three Hormones Actually Work in Your Body

To better understand this dance, consider how our cars work.

**The thyroid is like the gas pedal of a car.
It is the throttle for how fast the engine runs.**

The adrenals are two small pyramid-shaped glands, one above each kidney.

**In this car analogy, the adrenal is like the
steering wheel. It allows us to maneuver the turns
in the road and reach our destination.**

When a car is stopped, the steering wheel is not needed. When the car is moving along a simple straight road, it is hardly used. However, when the road bends or a sudden obstacle appears, it is instantly available for immediate corrective action.

This would be similar to the immediate increased energy provided by the adrenal for a fight-or-flight situation. Numerous energy chemicals allow the adrenals to provide additional alertness, tightness, tension, and focus for the sudden turns of confrontation or crisis.

Hormones produced by the sex glands (testes and ovaries) provide the spark for life. They are like turning on the ignition key, releasing the electricity to ignite the fuel. They control whether there is a charge or "spark" in one's life.

Sex hormones provide that extra oomph to send out pheromones, to magnetize the object of one's attraction, to help live out life's dreams. The spark of life is often generated via our reproductive hormones. Great music, great poetry, other works of genius and creativity, have arisen from the souls—and glands—of people who have used this spark productively.

Romance has clearly inspired some of our greatest novels and songs. This primal drive for reproduction is what makes animals fight for dominance, and inspires salmon to swim upstream. It is life longing for itself, the drive within living matter to perfect itself over generations. Your expression of your unique magnificence is a consequence of hormonal harmony.

RESTORING YOUR HORMONAL HARMONY

Understanding these principles can ensure success in whatever recommendations follow. Hopefully this will make your journey easier and richer.

This is the first day of the rest of your life!

The purpose of this first day and chapter is to help you to gain a more precise understanding of hormone balance, as well as to provide you with a simple useful model for these interacting systems. Tomorrow you will learn more about how and why your system has become unbalanced. Why is there all this disruption in what should be exquisite normal function?

The day after tomorrow, in chapter 3, you will assess your particular personal imbalance pattern by simple self-evaluations. This is what we call your apparent endo-type. Identifying this will help you to achieve better balance. You may confirm your actual endo-type by performing some simple home tests. Day Four is when you learn about and initiate the home testing process. (Receiving test results and interpretation will of course take longer than one day.)

In the meantime, finding your apparent endo-type via the self-evaluation questionnaires will allow you to take immediate supportive measures that can improve balance in your system right away. Day Five will encourage you to add these simple nutrients and exercises, along with adopting a mindset that will practically ensure success in your endeavors. Ideally, no Day Five suggestions would be implemented until after you have collected the samples for your baseline home tests.

The five-day jump start altogether is your first step toward healing. After these first five days of "jump start," you will be ready for the second step, of rebalancing tools as fully explained in chapters 6, 7, and 8, working first with whichever gland features most prominently in your symptoms. Once you have achieved your own measure of rebalance, you will be ready for continuing this success indefinitely with step three, long-term maintenance measures, as described in chapters 9 through 12.

Many people have temporary success with one program or another, only to backslide before long. This program can be totally different because it provides restorative measures that address the *root cause* of your problems.

With these three steps, you will have reset your thermostat, rebalanced your three-legged stool, and thus will be able to maintain your success and stamina far into the future.

We want to congratulate you on starting this first day. As Confucius said, "A journey of a thousand miles begins with a single step." Armed with this information, you will be ready for what follows. Our revealing and sometimes surprising self-evaluations await you.

But first, join us in the next chapter to learn more about *why* your system may have become unbalanced. This is vital; knowing how something became unbalanced is the first step toward being able to fix it properly.

You are now on your way to a fulfilling journey. In your hands, you are holding a clear and useful road map. Enjoy the trip.

CONCEPT SUMMARY

1. Consider that you may be one of many millions of Americans experiencing gland disruption.
2. Gland imbalance is very common, affecting at least one in every ten people in this country alone.
3. Most blood tests aren't sensitive enough to adequately reveal this level of problem. Your results can be normal, and you may still be affected by this situation.

ACTION SUMMARY

❑ If you have not been feeling your best, begin to write down what has been bothering you. (A written record will be of tremendous help later when you need to review it.)

❑ If you are tired of being overweight, dieting, and exercising to no avail, describe what you have tried to date and the results.

❑ If you are sick and tired of feeling frazzled, explain exactly how you feel when you're frazzled.

❑ If you can't even tell if your thinking is fuzzy or not, assume you may not be thinking clearly enough!

❑ Begin to organize your medical records.

❑ Call all offices of doctors you have seen, requesting copies of any information that could be related to these three glands.

❑ Ask them to fax or mail *actual test scores*, not just notes or a letter.

❑ Gather data about your unusual chemical exposures, early childhood illnesses, and any other previous diagnoses.

❑ Look for a possible endocrine connection.

❑ Document any unusual challenges with puberty, childbirth, menstruation, or menopause.

❑ List any difficulties in becoming pregnant or carrying to term.

❑ Describe any sexual difficulties or severe PMS symptoms.

❑ Seek out and chart relevant information about family history.

❑ Who has had diabetes or thyroid problems? Go back generations.

❑ Who had difficult childbirth, female problems, fertility or menstrual/menopausal challenges?

❑ Any cases of early gray hair? Mitral valve problems? Carpal tunnel syndrome? These can all be clues to gland imbalance.

❑ Are there any autoimmune issues (rheumatoid arthritis or other rheumatoid or immune difficulties)?

❑ Is there anything else that could implicate a possible gland imbalance?

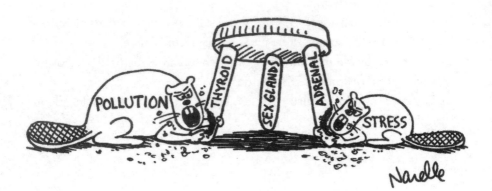

CHAPTER 2

DAY 2 OF YOUR JUMP START
DETERMINE THE CAUSE

I kept six honest serving men (they taught me all I knew): Their names were What and Why and When and How and Where and Who.

—Rudyard Kipling

Years ago, deep in the bowels of the earth, coal miners protected themselves from unseen poisonous gases by bringing a caged canary into the mine with them. The canary was notoriously sensitive to the toxic, invisible, odorless gases that often escaped from the coal seams, which could kill all the workers in the mine if not discovered early enough to allow for a hasty retreat to the surface. When the canary showed signs of distress, or actually keeled over, they knew it was time to evacuate.

All too often, the early signs of low-level poisoning take the form of increasing numbers of people feeling fat, fuzzy, or frazzled.

The most sensitive members of the human and animal populations are much like the canaries in the mines. They are the first to show distress, often becoming ill for unknown reasons. They provide the distant early warning for us all.

THE RAPIDLY GROWING "CANARY CLUB"

Many of us who are feeling fat, fuzzy, frazzled, or are plagued with various other symptoms have hormonal imbalance as their cause. Under normal circumstances these chemical messengers direct trillions of body cells to work together in harmony rather than chaos. Some of the most common complaints that people bring to doctor visits, when properly evaluated, are endocrine or metabolic in origin.

The 3-Legged Stool

Remember, the interplay of endocrine hormones constitutes the control system in charge of all body functions. Our hormones unify the other systems into a coherent, effective whole. The result can determine whether a person lives a full, vibrant life, or becomes a shadow of her potential self.

This grand hormonal-triad balance is like a three-legged stool. Each of these hormones affects the balance of the others. When any one of them is too low or too high, the stool is off balance.

Ideally we would strive to bring each leg of our three-legged "hormone stool" into proper range, ensuring a solid level base for the rest of our metabolic functions. Once these three are balanced, bodily activities such as weight distribution, memory recall, and emotional stability are improved.

The adrenals, for example, are involved in carbohydrate metabolism. Adrenal hormones affect pancreatic insulin levels, which facilitate the entry of sugar into cells. Adrenal secretions also help the liver to convert stored starch into readily available sugar. These adrenal hormones, called glucocorticoids, control much of our energy metabolism.

When this dance is off balance, you can have hypoglycemia, resulting in dramatic blood sugar drops that make you feel tired and irritable. The adrenal also produces mineralocorticoids, which control kidney function. When these adrenal hormones are off balance, you can retain too much water, causing ongoing bloating and puffiness.

> **While an imbalance of these crucial hormones can occasionally cause disastrous effects, it can more frequently cause milder difficulties—ones that can make you or loved ones feel fat, fuzzy, or frazzled.**

As a further example, the thyroid gland controls body temperature. If the gland output of thyroid hormone is low, your body temperature will be lower than normal, resulting in decreased metabolism. Slowed metabolism manifests clinically as digestive difficulties, uncomfortable blood-sugar fluctuations, decreased rate of wound healing, skin dryness, loss of hair, damaged nails, poor kidney function, and reduced muscle strength.

In addition, when the thyroid is low, other critical glands function more slowly, since thyroid hormone is essential to power most cells in the body. When adrenal function decreases, the result is excessive exhaustion, irritability, and insomnia. In women, decreased sex-hormone production can result in anything from mild PMS and low libido to endometriosis, infertility, miscarriage, and severe menopause symptoms. For men with lowered sex hormone, the result is often a sense of depression or bleakness, indecisiveness, and lowered libido, as well.

Women can go through menopause gracefully or experience great discomfort, depending upon the *balance* of the three-legged stool, not simply on estrogen alone—as has been previously promoted by the pharmaceutical industry. The difference between whether you have years of terrible symptoms (sometimes requiring antidepressants, sleeping pills, or memory-enhancing drugs) or a fairly uneventful transition depends on the proper balance of all three legs.

If your sex hormones are not balanced, you could experience sleep disturbance, depression, memory lapses, or lose your train of thought easily. In addition to these, and further serious complications, endocrine imbalance can also result in more subtle symptoms, difficult to diagnose and treat. While the scope of this condition is daunting, identifying the source is less so.

What could possibly be causing this situation? Why is it becoming increasingly common?

ENVIRONMENTAL POLLUTION: HORMONE-DISRUPTING FACTORS IN FOOD, AIR, AND WATER

For those who choose to look beyond the confines of standard medical practice, it is becoming increasingly clear that many of today's illnesses are a result of toxic accumulation in our bodies, as has likely never occurred before in human history. Recent studies have shown that even mothers' breast milk contains significant amounts of chemical pollutants taken into the body via the air, food, and water. Unfortunately, many of these stray chemicals cause hormone disruption.

This program specifically focuses on what *you* can do to decrease exposure to hormone-disrupting chemicals in your immediate environment. It then provides simple measures to *restore your glands* to health.

Whereas breast milk has been created by nature as the best and most perfect food for the new infant, the present chemical status of our surroundings is forcing us to reconsider how we live, how we procreate, and how we die. Worldwide, fertility rates are declining, a testament to this hormonal disruption.

Our biohormones are extremely potent, operating at concentrations so low that they can be measured only with the most sensitive analytical methods. For example, the estradiol (estrogen) that many women take in efforts to balance their sex hormones is active in concentrations of parts per *trillion*—rather than parts per million (or even parts per billion).

Levels of chemical contamination that would not be considered toxic in a laboratory study are nevertheless sufficient to create hormonal disruption in an adult, and in a child even more so. In utero, these same low levels can cause severe and permanent damage if the fetus is exposed to them at critical times of development. Though easily disrupted by minute doses of toxic chemicals, these hormones are nonetheless crucial to who we are. In fact, their balance dictates how we mature.

You could become fat, fuzzy, or frazzled from exposure
to synthetic chemicals at concentrations much lower
than would generally be considered poisonous or toxic.

In addition to normal daily function, normal growth and development depend on getting just the right hormone message, in exactly the right amount, to just the right place—at the right time. In utero or in growing children, missing the "cue" (the right stimulus at the right time), can result in lifelong problems. Similarly, adding a disrupting foreign substance to the system at specific times of growth can also have lifelong impact.

DES: A Notorious Example of the Synthetic Hormone Problem

Diethylstilbestrol (DES) was a pharmaceutical drug supplied years ago to more than 5 million women, purportedly to prevent miscarriages. Developed in the 1930s and heavily promoted in the 1950s, DES was the first synthetic estrogen created, and considered a miracle breakthrough. At that time, people thought many problems were due to lack of estrogen. DES was given in pregnancy to prevent miscarriage and premature birth, to suppress milk production after childbirth, to alleviate hot flashes after menopause, to treat acne, even as a morning-after contraceptive for young women. It was also used in livestock to fatten the animals. Yet, despite the high hopes it engendered, the substance created a terrible disaster.

Amazingly, it didn't directly harm the mothers who were given this drug. Instead, it affected their developing babies, leaving them with lifelong major problems. It ruined their chances for becoming pregnant and caused rare cancers in millions of young women. It wasn't until years later that *the New England Journal of Medicine* published a paper showing the correlation between mothers taking DES and daughters being affected by cancer.

It now appears that DES-exposed women also have a greater likelihood of developing autoimmune diseases, such as Hashimoto's thyroiditis and Grave's disease, as well as other rheumatoid problems. People with mild versions of these illnesses commonly have problems with their weight, memory, or emotions. In other words, while some victims of chemical exposure develop full-blown autoimmune diseases, others might have the "milder" version of simply being fat, fuzzy, or frazzled.

It is very clear that the human body can mistake a human-made chemical for a hormone, disrupting normal hormone action.

This entire DES episode was a tragic and unintended chapter in our history. A recent book, *The Greatest Experiment Ever Performed on Women*, by Barbara Seaman, sheds further light on a recurrent pattern of the medical and pharmaceutical industries, that of pushing lucrative estrogen preparations into women's bodies. Clearly evidence has shown that these estrogenic compounds can potentially cause harm for generations to come, disrupting the developing human with consequences that may defy current diagnosis. We suggest, in addition, that some of the estrogen overuse is behind today's fat, fuzzy, and frazzled epidemic.

Since we live in an environment increasingly filled with chemicals that interfere with our natural hormone function, it may be many years or even decades before a fuller understanding of the impact of this chemical cascade can be reviewed. For now, we can be aware of potential harm and act accordingly in our own best interests.

We therefore join the chorus of other scientists concerned about this environmental connection, recommending what is known as the precautionary principle. This wise advice suggests that when an activity potentially raises the threat of harm to the health of humans or the environment, cautionary steps should be taken *even* if the cause-and-effect relationship has not yet been fully demonstrated.

It is becoming increasingly apparent that we are slowly being flooded by a massive wave of endocrine disruption. Some of the long-term effects of these increased chemical exposures include infertility, predisposition to cancer, and, most commonly, the symptoms of disordered metabolism.

We concur with ecologist Sandra Steingraber, MD, in her recent books on the topic, that those individuals or industries involved in promoting potentially harmful activity should be held accountable for proving that their actions are *not* causing harm, rather than allowing the public to be exposed to possible danger. Industrial pollutants are the major offenders in many of these health issues. We therefore call for greater governmental oversight, with informed and democratic process, in ensuring that industry acts responsibly in the creation, research, and use of its products. In the meanwhile, however, we provide information to enable you to remain healthy!

This country is no exception to the alarming worldwide decrease in sperm counts and increase in male impotency noted in recent years. (Consider the huge sales of Viagra as a possible indicator of this phenomenon.) Global reports of striking deformities in sex organs and mating behaviors of birds, frogs, fish, and mammals have—until recently—confounded the scientists.

Our best researchers, with three decades of painstaking evaluation, are now reporting that many widely used synthetic chemicals, including insecticides, plasticizers, and electric components previously considered safe are actually causing devastating hormonal chaos. The striking increase in environmental hormone-disrupting chemicals parallels the striking rise in hormone-related illness in humans. We are in the midst of a hormonal epidemic; this could well be affecting you. Indeed, this issue goes far beyond DES and other intentional hormone-active substances.

DDT: An "Accidental" Hormone

DES is merely the first synthetic estrogen marketed as a drug. Other synthetic estrogens have been discovered only after the fact, for they were first created to be insecticides! The most notorious example of this phenomenon is the now-banned chemical DDT, lauded as a fantastic breakthrough, and certainly deadly on the insect population. In retrospect, it is curious that scientists could consider a chemical so deadly to insects to be harmless to humans.

Only years later was DDT found to mimic the effect of estrogen in the body, first observed in laboratory tests of roosters exposed to DDT.

The roosters became feminized, looking and acting like hens. Gradually, over decades, further experimentation confirmed this finding in humans, as well. Eventually the substance was banned from use, but not before billions of tons of DDT were widely distributed in the environment. The concern is that DDT is a persistent chemical. Banning its use is very much like locking the barn door after the horse has run away.

Not only does every animal on the planet now show traces of DDT stored in its fat, but also the concentration in human mothers' milk currently approaches levels toxic enough to suggest that some breast milk should not be fed to babies.

Today there are tens of thousands of chemicals in wide usage whose possible hormone-disrupting effects have not been evaluated.

PCBs: Considered Innocuous, Proved Otherwise

Another notorious example is polychlorinated biphenyls (PCBs). PCBs were developed as insulation material in electrical equipment. It was not known at the time that this rather innocuous chemical, also used as a flame retardant, had serious hormone-disrupting effects. It happens to be another extremely persistent chemical in the environment, and is now widely distributed throughout the ecosphere, in every state of the union, to the most distant deserts, and into polar regions. Just as with DDT, the supposedly innocuous PCBs have recently been found to exist in high levels in human breast milk.

What this might mean for you is that the amount of PCBs in your body right now could be enough to throw off your delicate hormonal balance. Once you know this, however, you can take corrective action to remedy this situation. For instance, if the PCB disruption in your body is reducing your thyroid function, you can counter that with some simple vitamin or herbal medicine to increase your thyroid hormone production.

The Dioxin Dilemma

Here's yet another example. In the realm of synthetic chemicals, dioxin is one of the most notorious substances. In contradistinction to previous chemicals we have discussed, dioxin was not created intentionally. It is an inadvertent by-product; a contaminant created during the manufacture of other chemicals, like pesticides and wood preservatives, also occurring in the burning of plastics.

There are close to a hundred different variants in the dioxin chemical family, including those that contaminated the notorious Agent Orange, used in the Vietnam War as a defoliant.

Like DDT and PCBs, dioxin is a very persistent chemical in the environment. It is similarly fat-loving, accumulating in the adipose tissues of our bodies. Like DDT and PCBs, it has been detected virtually everywhere on the planet.

Perhaps of wider import than any of its other effects is the ability of dioxin to interfere with hormone levels in the body. In animal studies, rats given dioxin experienced decreased testosterone levels and decrease in the size of various sex organs. It appeared to affect sexual behavior in males born to mothers given dioxin, as well as showing a decrease in sperm count by as much as 40 percent.

It appears that dioxin acts as a powerful and persistent hormone, capable of producing major changes at very low levels. Most intriguing is that these animal studies found significant effects at levels of dioxin to which humans were exposed regularly.

Water Fluoridation: The Twentieth Century's Greatest Advance . . . or Worst Mistake?

One of the most well-meaning and honored scientific traditions in this country has been the addition of fluoride to municipal water supplies for the prevention of tooth decay. The outgoing Surgeon General of the United States at the turn of the millennium heralded this maneuver as one of the top ten health achievements of the twentieth century.

However, like some of the above-mentioned substances previously thought to be innocuous, fluoride is beginning to show its true colors. This substance, touted as harmless, has been used by the medical profession in the past to slow down the activity of overactive thyroid glands. It is no longer used medically for this purpose since the development of better medicines, propylthiouracil (PTU), and methemazole (Tapazole). However, as a result of its ability to slow thyroid function, fluoride has systemic effects, as well.

Long before fluoride was used in drinking water, its industrial application was known to be hazardous to exposed workers, who are still required to adopt serious precautionary procedures for handling toxic chemicals. When in contact with fluoride, these include wearing full protective suits, eye covers, gloves, and facial masks. The substance's disposal has long been known to be hazardous to farm animals and crops, resulting in decreased plant growth and health hazards to exposed creatures.

The original research performed to prove the benefits of fluoride on teeth studied naturally occurring sodium fluoride (NaF) on research animals. However, this is *not* what is being added to public water supplies today. Instead, what is being used to artificially fluoridate public waters is hydrofluosilicic acid, an industrial waste product of the fertilizer and aluminum industries.

With scientific evidence mounting against this practice, many more nations are rejecting it. Less than 5 percent of the world's population drinks artificially fluoridated water (most naturally occurring water has some sodium fluoride), and in Europe it is only 2 percent. A number of countries have banned fluoridation, including Japan, Denmark, Sweden, India, and Holland.

In our country, virtually all the 1,500 scientists, engineers, and lawyers of the EPA headquarters in Washington, D.C., unanimously stood against fluoridation through their professional employees union. To read their letter, go to www.fluoridealert.org or www.keepersofthewell.com.

What Does This All Mean?

Examples from across the globe, in animals and humans, have pointed to a troubling trend. What appears to be hormonal disruption is affecting the fish, the birds, and the animals. The imbalance affects their behavior, not just their reproduction. Humans are not exempt from this phenomenon. Hormonal disruption, for us, can take many forms. In a small number of people, it can be a dramatic and lifelong difficulty. In a much larger number of people, however, it can be more subtle, causing diffi-culties with weight, mental focus, or mood.

If you are challenged by feeling fat, fuzzy, or frazzled, or by similar ongoing symptoms that have been hard to diagnose and treat, you can deal with this situation most effectively once you acknowledge the possi-bility of toxic exposure as a factor in your symptoms.

Some of the most common, ordinary, and frustrating daily life conditions have this silent epidemic of glandular disruption as their hidden cause.

- If you have spent years with yo-yo dieting, where nothing seems to work for very long, this information may change your life.
- If you have had memory or focus challenges, interfering with your ability to be effective, this book can help.
- If your nerves are constantly on edge, making you jumpy, ir-ritable, or anxious, perhaps unable to sleep well, we have some answers.
- If you have been plagued by multiple discomforts, or even one uncomfortable persistent symptom, it could be metabolic in origin.
- If you feel like a shadow of your former self, and aren't sure why, this new diagnosis could be life altering.

HEREDITY AND STRESS: MAJOR *INTERNAL* CAUSES OF HORMONE IMBALANCE

Environmental factors are not solely responsible for this massive epi-demic of hormone imbalance. Other contributing factors to the fat, fuzzy, and frazzled epidemic come from within, be they genetic or stress related.

Hereditary Factors

Some people have low adrenal function for the same reason that others have low thyroid function, or diabetes. They inherit a tendency for their immune system to disrupt their hormone-producing glands. Autoim-mune illness occurs when the body starts attacking itself erroneously.

This bizarre activity warrants much greater medical attention, given that autoimmune illnesses have increased dramatically in recent years. It is the third major category of illness in the United States, where 50 million Americans suffer from some kind of autoimmune condition.

Most commonly discussed is the situation of immune impairment of the islets of Langerhans cells in the pancreas, resulting in type 1 diabetes wherein less insulin is being produced, making less insulin available for the vital process of facilitating the transport of sugar into the cells.

Less well known, but actually much more common in occurrence, is the situation wherein the inherited autoimmune tendency results in impairment of the thyroid-hormone producing cells, called Hashimoto's thyroiditis. This causes the thyroid gland to secrete a diminished amount of T3 and T4 thyroid hormones, together essential for the body functions of temperature regulation, energy production, growth, and development, among others.

Even less recognized than the cases above is the immune-caused decrease in adrenal gland hormone output, including cortisol and cortisone for handling extended stress, adrenaline for dealing with immediate stress, aldosterone for maintaining salt–fluid balance and stable blood pressure, to name just a few.

A severe version of this decreased adrenal hormone production is called Addison's disease, a condition that plagued President John F. Kennedy during his presidency. Most cases of Addison's are autoimmune in origin, but researchers tell us that the number of people diagnosed with Addison's is just the tip of a very large iceberg of people who have a *milder* version of adrenal insufficiency. Common symptoms include low blood pressure; low blood sugar, causing mood and energy shifts after eating; exaggerated responses to stress; severe difficulty getting going in the morning; and extreme irritability.

Emily knew that she was pushing her luck when she agreed to make multiple huge life changes all at the same time, including relocating several states away, while also taking on more responsibility as a manager. She had always been ambitious, pushing herself to be near the top of her class in high school and college. In fact, she became ill with mononucleosis in her last year of college, evidently from being so worn down.

She knew even prior to her move to San Francisco that she had become short-tempered in recent months, and more apt to lose her cool at work. Although still in her twenties, she pushed herself hard, driven as if she had much to accomplish and never enough time. Her particular body response was to become increasingly irritable.

Upon leaving our office the day she met Phoebe and Meredith, she had handed each of them her business card and suggested that maybe they could stay in touch. They all exchanged numbers and seemed to feel connected despite their symptomatic differences.

Though the other women were older than she, Emily had not met many friendly people in her new area, and she felt a bond with Phoebe and Meredith. Since her mother was far away, and seriously ill with rheumatoid arthritis, Emily appreciated having the chance to talk with these women, who might be in a position to support her through this lonely time. At work, many of her colleagues were not friendly to her, though perhaps this was less a reflection on Emily than of themselves and their own frustrations.

Emily, as an only child, felt obligated to help with her sick mother, but she resented this long-distance burden. Accepting this new position had allowed her the perfect escape, freeing her to spread her own wings after years as a caregiver and to insist that others help out more.

At times, when alone, Emily felt despondent, wondering how she could ever create a life for herself while working so hard. She enjoyed her stretching class, which she hoped would prevent arthritis, but that was hardly the place she would meet people her own age, as most participants were seniors.

Phoebe, estranged from her daughter, who was Emily's age, enjoyed the welcome addition of Emily in her life.

Meredith had two young teens, and a younger sister, who looked like Emily and had similar mannerisms. Fortuitously, the three women clicked. The week after they met, Emily was feeling especially down. Coming across Meredith's number by the phone in the hall, she called Meredith to see if she wanted to meet for tea.

They enjoyed learning more about each other's lives. Emily had received ideas from our clinic to help her get started in feeling better, but she was waiting for results of her testing before making any major changes.

As they sipped tea, Emily cried about her mother's arthritis and diabetes. Meredith listened attentively, allowing Emily to talk about this for the first time since her move.

"Rheumatoid arthritis and diabetes are both autoimmune conditions," Meredith told Emily. "It's great that you're working with someone to begin to deal with that aspect now. I have similar situations in my immediate family, but only recently learned that what I'm going through is also autoimmune illness. I've been working with Dr. Shames on this for a while, and I'm amazed at how little I knew at first!"

If you or one of your friends or family has the genetic tendency to make antibodies against the adrenal gland, you may well be functioning with a subadequate amount of one or more adrenal hormones. This means that you would be moving through life as an **emotional** (adrenal) endo-type, *unless* you take corrective action that can reduce or completely alleviate the situation. The same holds true for autoimmune low-thyroid or autoimmune sex-gland disruption.

The Secret Relationship: Autoimmunity and Environment

One of the main reasons for uncomfortable aging is the lack of careful medical attention given to mild or moderate autoimmune glandular conditions.

Part of the reason that many people continue to feel fat, fuzzy, and frazzled is that doctors often do not diagnose adrenal, thyroid, or sex-gland abnormality, *except in the most severe cases.*

For this reason, many people, perhaps even you, are attempting to live normally with underfunctioning gland output, causing you to live only half a life.

There is a crucial relationship between the chemical disruption described in the beginning of this chapter and the autoimmune phenomenon. *The people most sensitive to the devastating effects of environmental pollutants are those genetically prone to autoimmunity.* It is very inheritable, so check your family history for diabetes, thyroid, or rheumatoid problems.

Toxic exposure, even in small amounts, is known to trigger a latent and underlying autoimmune condition. Although there are other triggers, such as injuries, infections, bereavement, puberty, childbirth, and menopause, the chemical connection is a major one. Recent research cited in *Our Stolen Future*, by Theo Colborn, et al., points to this environmental trigger connection as a primary cause of much of this kind of illness in people genetically at risk.

External toxins, however, are not the only cause of gland disruption, simply the most relevant *external* reason. Another predominant or major cause of gland disruption is *internal*: stress.

The Stress Connection

In chapter 7, we explain in greater detail how the stress of modern life raises hormone levels, particularly cortisol, causing multiple symptoms, including high blood pressure, increased heart rate, an uncomfortable sense of urgency rather than calm. In fact, the scientist who popularized the concept of stress, Hans Selye, MD, described in his blockbuster book *The Stress of Life* how this "stress response" negatively impacts related organs and various systems.

Life is dramatically complicated today. In earlier times, a stress was an immediate fight-or-flight situation, either facing off with another caveman, or running from a saber-toothed tiger. Our bodily responses to stress are relatively unchanged since those early times, but now the stressors are different. Due to the complex nature of fast-paced living, we can spend weeks (or even months), engaged in chronic, ongoing tension and anxiety. Long-term projects can take months of effort. Mounting concern about whether deadlines or expectations will be met can wreak havoc on our bodies. Having to function quickly in certain life-or-death situations, particularly involving traffic, can keep our cortisol raised to unnatural levels for prolonged periods of time, causing depletion.

When we are constantly faced with chronic ongoing stress and exhaustion, our chemical mechanisms try to handle this as they would in the face of sudden dramatic confrontation. There is no caveman to fight with a club, rarely a tiger to escape from, yet we still engage our fight-or-flight responses, sometimes continuously. This causes a severe and unprecedented chemical flooding of the body with stress chemicals that seem to have been intended for much more episodic and short-lived problems, leaving the glands that produce them unable to keep pace with the continuous need for hormone production.

The fight-or-flight chemicals are our adrenal hormones. One of the major ones is adrenaline, also called epinephrine. Its main function is for instantaneous response to threat. Adrenaline comes from the inner core of the adrenal gland, its release activated directly by fast-firing nerves from the brain.

Another chemical is cortisol, also from the adrenal gland. Its main purpose is to handle longer-term stress situations. Cortisol is produced in the outer cortex of the adrenal gland, and is activated by hormone control from the pituitary, a much slower but more enduring process.

There are other adrenal hormones, but these two constitute the basic paradigm for short-term and longer-acting adrenal function. The problem is that continued high secretion of adrenaline over extended periods wears the body out. If you are not actually fighting or running away, it makes you very jumpy and nervous to have massive amounts of adrenaline or cortisol flowing in your bloodstream. The muscles remain tight, resulting in more aches and pains, and minor injuries from daily activity. The mind stays on red alert, causing a decrease in restorative sleep, the time generally used for good maintenance and repair.

To make matters worse, long-term excess cortisol levels actually wear down body structures, disintegrating their cell membranes. For example, it has long been known that high levels of cortisol result in "stress ulcers" of the digestive tract. All of this is akin to a car that is always being driven at excessively high speed and high temperatures. Things wear out more quickly at this pace, especially due to lack of proper maintenance. The parts of this car are likely to fail more readily than would those of a well-attended vehicle.

Eventually, the adrenal gland is not able to keep up with the production demands of such a high-stress life. The symptoms of adrenal insufficiency can include dark circles under the eyes, low blood pressure, lack of libido, weakness, allergies, muscle and joint pains, dry skin, cystic breasts, difficulty recuperating from respiratory illness, anxiety, tendency to startle easily, depression, premature aging, and reduced stamina for confrontation.

Thus, your best protection against these internal and external ravages is to recognize the problem and take corrective action.

Our next chapter provides a few simple self-evaluations to help you determine what type of endocrine challenge may be foremost in your own situation. Armed with this knowledge, you can then perform some simple home tests to confirm your endo-type, which then allows you to proceed quickly and efficiently to reclaim your total health.

CONCEPT SUMMARY

1. Some of the most common complaints that people bring to doctor visits, when properly evaluated, are endocrine/metabolic in origin.
2. This hormonal dance is like a grand three-legged stool. Each of these hormones affects the balance of this basic hormonal triad. When any gland production is too low or too high the stool is off balance.
3. Gland imbalance has two major causes:
   External (synthetic chemicals in the environment acting as hormone disruptors)
   Internal (hormone disruption combined with the pace and stress of modern life to cause a flooding of biochemicals that negatively impact gland function)
4. The concentration of chemicals that can cause hormone disruption is *much* less than that considered toxic by regulatory agencies!
5. A large contributor to the epidemic of fat, fuzzy, and frazzled is hormone disruption caused by environmental pollution.
6. A more internal source of hormone imbalance derives from our glandular response to the extreme and ongoing stress of modern life, coupled with genetic tendencies toward autoimmunity.

7. The solution for hormone imbalance is to first reduce your exposure to toxic chemicals, including those in certain foods, then to nourish your glands to create better balance.

8. What has frequently been neglected is the importance of considering *all three major regulatory hormones* in any rebalancing effort. This program specifically addresses that concern.

ACTION SUMMARY

(Note: These will be thoroughly discussed in greater detail in further related chapters.)

❑ Eat less chemical-laden and more organic foods whenever possible. Especially, find meat and poultry that is hormone-free.

❑ Strive to make your home and workplace as chemical-free as possible. Use natural cleaning products in your home.

❑ Switch from neurotoxic chemical perfumes/fragrance sprays (personal and household), substituting natural organic essential oils.

❑ Use HEPA air filters in your sleeping and workspace when possible, and crack a window when sleeping.

❑ Instead of tap water, drink filtered water, particularly water treated by reverse osmosis when in fluoridated communities.

❑ Stop hiring pest control companies to spray your house or lawn.

❑ Try to spend less time in areas near billowing smokestacks or near other massive air pollution, wherever you can smell fumes.

❑ Become more involved with stress reduction, working to reduce the sources (what makes you uptight) and finding ways to reduce your negative responses (more exercise, reflective meditation).

❑ Avoid spending time with vexing people whenever possible.

❑ Direct your immune system to help your glands function well. Visualize your system restoring balance easily throughout the day.

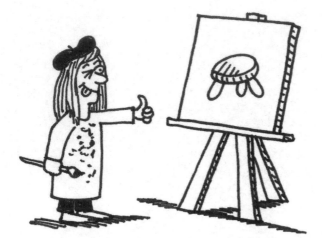

CHAPTER 3

DAY 3 OF YOUR JUMP START
ESTIMATE YOUR ENDO-TYPE
USING SELF-EVALUATIONS

Here am I, dying of a hundred good symptoms.
—Alexander Pope

Phoebe was forty-six when she first began to experience mild occasional hot flashes. By age forty-eight, these had grown into uncomfortable heat surges that forced her to drop whatever she was doing and cool down fast. Her gynecologist put her on estrogen, which made the hot flashes less bothersome, but caused other things to worsen.

She began to feel more sluggish, with uncomfortable constipation and very dry skin. Also upsetting was her now-increasing hair loss. Most disturbing, however, was her accelerating weight gain. For the last six months, she had been averaging a weight gain of three pounds per month.

*After she consulted with us, we suggested she take the self-evaluations provided in this chapter. Sure enough, Phoebe's main score was indicative of the (low-thyroid) **physical** endo-type. When she elected to then perform the home testing presented in chapter 4 to confirm this apparent endo-type, she was indeed low thyroid. The extra sensitive home tests showed low, despite her standard, doctor-ordered blood test being normal. This suggested that Phoebe may have had a long-standing undetected thyroid problem.*

We told Phoebe that a mild low-thyroid situation often masquerades as severe menopause, and that taking estrogen can accelerate an underlying low-thyroid condition. When Phoebe was further tested for the binding proteins that are increased by estrogen, they were, in fact, high. Phoebe's thyroid hormone was primarily caught in her blood-stream, allowing less to get into her tissues. The result was that Phoebe now had a lower metabolic rate.

According to her other doctors, her blood tests looked like she had plenty of thyroid hormone. This was true—but when the more impor-tant tissue *levels were taken into account via the home tests, Phoebe was shown to be a low thyroid person. Because of the estrogen effect, her thyroid tissue level was now even lower, causing her weight gain and hair loss amid normal blood tests.*

This situation was making Phoebe crazy. She knew that some-thing was not right. The doctor had even increased her estrogen to try to fix things, leaving her feeling worse. The doctor was frustrated, she was frustrated, and those around her were affected.

Again, through Phoebe, we see the importance of looking at all three energy hormones all at once, not just one at a time. The doctor measured the amount of thyroid in Phoebe's bloodstream and said she was fine. Very few doctors today check basal temperatures or ankle re-flexes, long-standing ways to evaluate thyroid function. Most physicians now rely totally on blood tests, which, as you can see, are sometimes misleading. Often, a more accurate picture of one's hormone status can come from saliva tests, which evaluate actual tissue levels, rather than what is in the bloodstream.

Many people who are on thyroid medication and who also take es-trogen for menopause or even birth control end up needing *more* thyroid medicine because of the estrogen-binding effect. As long as the thyroid situation is understood, estrogen can be taken comfortably when neces-sary; however, it's important to note that often estrogen is not as nec-essary for a patient's comfort when the thyroid is well balanced.

**Awareness of the status of all three glands is
crucial to proper balancing of any one of them.**

Looking at all these glands together as a composite when adjusting any one of them will give you better perspective, and a better end result.

Menopause, like puberty and childbirth, is one of many important hormonal transitions where finding a comfortable balance becomes especially important, and where more than one hormone needs to be considered. Males have a form of this situation also during their midlife years, called andropause, which can bring various low-energy symptoms. It may seem like depression, and without careful evaluation, it is often incorrectly treated as depression, an incomplete approach at best.

General times of transition—such as relocation of home or office, of children or spouses—affect us very deeply on many levels, predominantly emotionally, which can result in burnt-out adrenals. Complicating these changes are the ones that are natural and hormonal, including puberty, childbirth, and menopause. This is because hormonal influences are additive and cumulative. Even accidents and trauma can cause a shift in the hormone balance.

EXPLORING THE ENDO-TYPE MODEL

Why look at hormones? Because the hormones grease the wheels of our machinery. They come into contact with every part of our bodies, directing the operation of the cells and organs.

The traditional medical approach would be to treat your (or Phoebe's) individual symptoms, so that if you were having a chronic skin condition, you may end up being sent to a dermatologist, who might provide you with some medicine to stop the skin problem. However, if what was *causing* this skin problem was related to a hormone imbalance, you may experience a temporary relief by removing the symptom, only to find that other symptoms become more pronounced. The reason for this is that you need a systemic fix, not just a symptom fix.

As Western practitioners, we have joined a growing cadre of professionals who seek a deeper understanding of the cause of dis-ease, in order to effect long-term healing. We believe in a body-mind-spirit approach, which allows for integrated restoration of full function. Enhancing the healing power of our bodies by restoring balance, we can enjoy lasting freedom from many of the most bothersome physical, mental, and emotional conditions.

**The endo-type model allows you to determine
which of your three main energy glands is *currently*
the predominant culprit in causing your problems.**

In other words, even if you have multigland involvement, you can start immediately to tackle the challenges of your main gland. Is it physical (thyroid), mental (sex hormones), or emotional (adrenal)?

Why do we name them this way? While each of these three glands can affect you physically, emotionally, and mentally, the thyroid's impact is *predominantly* physical. The sex glands have a major impact on our thinking, while the adrenals largely wreak havoc with emotions. By working on your primary glandular problem first, you are paving the way for less discomfort and more strength to tackle other possible cofactors. Working in this stepwise manner, you should be able to enjoy more time every day, while building a foundation for good health for the rest of your life.

The **Physical** Endo-Type

If your primary gland problem is thyroid, you are a **physical** endo-type. Those who have thyroid problems know that it can make you feel depressed, and can imbalance you in many other ways. But we have chosen to call the person whose major gland imbalance is in the thyroid **physical** endo-type, largely because this is the arena where most symptoms are found. Thyroid sufferers can have a laundry list of symptoms (see chapter 6), most affecting the body itself.

The **Mental** Endo-Type

If your primary gland affected is sex glands, you are a **mental** endo-type. **Mental** endo-types often have as a presenting symptom the inability to focus, think clearly, or remember well. For this reason, we recommend working on the mental plane, using specific vitamins, minerals, herbs, foods, and mental exercises that are known to boost mental powers.

The **Emotional** Endo-Type

If adrenal is your main presenting gland, you are the **emotional** endo-type. People with adrenal as the predominant gland causing problems can be very nervous, anxious, jittery, irritable, angry, or otherwise emotionally unstable. The adrenal is meant to deal with fight-or-flight issues, and when affected, can make the person's entire life feel like a roller coaster, alternating between these high-energy modes. Both can burn you out, leaving you absolutely depleted, after long periods of irritable behavior. The **emotional** endo-types aren't having fun often, and neither are the people around them!

If you have more than one of these three major glands affected, which many people do, you will derive great benefit from first balancing your primary gland. You may not need to do anything further, or you may later want to feel even better by putting focused attention on your other glands. You will find that balancing your primary gland, or endo-type, can allow you to begin to feel so much like your old, healthier self that you can *then* more easily take better care of yourself to feel your best.

The identification of your main gland causing problems is what we are referring to as your *primary or predominant* endo-type. Working directly with that gland can often allow you to feel better fast.

WHY LEARN ABOUT YOUR ENDO-TYPE?

Remember Meredith from chapter 1, who had abnormal sex-gland hormone levels, leading to fuzzy thinking? It seemed her memory problem became more severe after taking birth control pills, but she didn't know what to do about it. She had wondered if taking more estrogen was really a good idea, and hoped to find some other way to normalize her periods that would help—rather than hurt—her mental function.

Her prescribing doctor's advice? Her residual fuzzy-thinking problem must be due to something else. Later, after the problem intensified, she consulted with us and took the self-evaluation question-

*naires, which gave her a high estrogen point score due to several of her long-standing issues, suggesting that she was a **mental** endo-type. We told her we would be able to recommend a different intervention if the home tests confirmed this apparent endo-type.*

Meredith is not alone in this situation. As we age, our glands begin to show signs of slowing down, or malfunctioning. Normal life transitions, coupled with years of exposures to gland-altering chemicals in the environment, begin to take their toll in vague and nondescript ways that can result in personality changes. It becomes difficult to tell what is causing what, as symptoms mount to undermine health. Many health challenges occur around puberty, childbirth, menopause, or trauma, as well as during times of major stress and change, leaving us confused as to how to begin to tackle the web of discomfort.

For these reasons, it can be life-altering for you to uncover your endo-type. It can prevent wasted years that might otherwise be enjoyable and incredibly productive.

If you are too high or low in one of your major regulatory hormones, endo-type evaluation will reveal this, offering a road map to correct it.

Consider yet another example of why knowing your endo-type can help.

Recall Emily, the twenty-nine-year-old stockbroker who had for years been working full throttle, at high energy, yet was feeling anxious. Even a friend had told her to get her adrenals checked.

Before consulting with us, she took the advice of a nutritionist, who suggested 25 mg of dehydroepiandro-sterone (DHEA) for adrenal support. This over-the-counter adrenal precursor, rather than help her stress symptoms, resulted in the development of adult acne, excessive breast tenderness, and annoying water retention. Had she and her nutritionist known more about her endo-type, they could have selected a different adrenal support, one that would not further increase her (already high) reproductive hormones. For Emily, a better choice at that time might have been pregnenolone, which helps in the production of cortisol. The DHEA does little for cortisol, and instead might increase estrogen and testosterone, which Emily did not need at all.

- First, it helps to know if your fat, fuzzy, or frazzled problem is because of hormonal imbalance, and if so, to what degree. Is it a mild or a major factor? You can do better if you first answer these questions, rather than taking a shot in the dark, possibly causing further imbalance or muddying the picture, making eventual balance even more difficult.
- Next, it is crucial to understand *which hormone* is most unbalanced and needs correction first. How can you fix something if you don't know what's wrong?
- How your three major hormones line up is the crux of the matter, however. This is our main contention. These three regulatory hormones do not work in isolation from one another. You cannot adjust any one of them effectively without taking them all into account.

Adjusting any one of these hormones affects the other two. You may now create another imbalance that must be considered.

This is what went wrong when our menopausal friend Phoebe was simply given estrogen (a common practice until the recent warnings against it from the Women's Health Initiative). This is also what went wrong when Meredith was given thyroid, as well as when Emily took DHEA. Each of these corrections might have been a good idea in isolation, but in the presence of a coexisting hormone imbalance, they caused further disruption.

Knowing your endo-type can help you to make better choices that nurture your wellness, avoiding situations that contribute to illness. The choices you make are a result of the time and focus you give to them, and they can be a reflection of your belief systems and life patterns.

HOW TO USE YOUR SYMPTOMS TO DETERMINE YOUR ENDOCRINE PROFILE

How do you find out if you're low in any one component of this three-gland system? How can you really tell? Most people imagine that if they were at risk for having a hormone abnormality, their doctor would tell them after running some well-chosen blood tests.

While this is a reasonable expectation, it rarely happens. In reality, the questionnaire method from this chapter may actually be more useful to you than a doctor visit, especially if you don't yet have a practitioner who is competent to advise you in this arena.

There are two main reasons that may prevent you from receiving an accurate diagnosis readily.

- First, many women depend on gynecologists for help in these situations. Gynecologists are trained to look for surgical ways to intervene; they are not trained as endocrine specialists. So what about the endocrinologists, who *are* trained in this way? Because of the currently enormous number of people with diabetes, many endocrinologists are generally too occupied with diabetic management to give people who are merely fat, fuzzy, or frazzled the attention they deserve.
- Those endocrinologists who *are* interested in hormonal challenges beyond diabetes are often totally focused on standard blood test results. These determinations, although taken as gospel, are in reality not nearly so effective as the scientists would like, or as many physicians believe them to be.

Blood tests generally do not measure the actual level of bioavailable hormone in your tissues.

The hormones we're discussing in this book, as we have said, are carried in the blood, tightly bound to special proteins. Only a very small percentage (often a tiny fraction of 1 percent) is free to disperse into the tissues to do its work. The blood tests don't easily measure this free hormone. Instead, they usually identify the total concentration in the blood, an inaccurate measure of how much active free hormone is really available to work for you. The blood tests are not as sensitive, or as relevant, as they need to be.

At medical schools, the best medical professors teach their students that a well-taken medical history is often much more valuable than physical exams and lab tests combined. However, the time constraints of managed care mean that the careful focused history performed by the well-trained practitioner is becoming a thing of the past.

Nowadays, this initial evaluation is often relegated to a questionnaire that a person fills out prior to coming to see the doctor. The problem with some of these forms is that they are not sufficiently detailed or focused enough to make subtle hormonal distinctions of the sort that we are telling you may be very important for your health and well-being. The result is that some of the most important questions about your symptoms end up not being asked.

In the symptom questions below, we try to correct that shortcoming. A careful evaluation of your symptoms is a major contribution to solving the puzzle of your health. Be sure to share this information with your health provider. Together, the two of you can make the best use of this hormone data.

SELF-EVALUATIONS

Determine Your Apparent Endo-Type

This section will give you a good idea of what might be your predominant endo-type. Here you will find a simple evaluation for each gland, which will help determine whether you are too high or too low in that gland's main hormone. Everyone should answer every question of every evaluation below, except those labeled as specific for the other sex.

These related endocrine glands have several symptoms in common. Don't be concerned if you answer yes for the same symptoms on more than one evaluation. This will be taken into account during the scoring phase. The ultimate goal is to help you ascertain which is your predominant endo-type.

Guidelines for Responding to Self-Evaluations

- When answering these questions, give yourself zero (0) points if you do not have this symptom, or if the question does not apply to you at all.
- Give yourself 1 point if the symptom is *noticeable* (i.e., you're aware of it, but not particularly bothered).
- Give 2 points if it's *annoying* (i.e., you're frequently aware of it, and bothered by its presence.)
- Give 3 points if it's *limiting* (i.e., it's definitely compromising your life in some important way).

The first four questions of each section are starred, and **set in bold-face,** because they are most important. Therefore, give them DOUBLE whatever would be their usual point score.

(For example, on the first test below, for low thyroid, if you have had problems with weight, and it's "annoying," that would ordinarily be 2 points. But because the usual point score is doubled for questions marked with asterisks, give yourself *4* points.)

THYROID GLAND EVALUATIONS

A. Could You Be LOW Thyroid? Do You Have the Following?

1. ***DOUBLE SCORE* Problems with weight (very easy to gain, OR extremely hard to lose, despite sensible food intake AND good exercise)?** _____ × 2 = _____
2. ***DOUBLE SCORE* Problems with body temperature (feeling chilly when others don't OR cold feet and/or hands OR needing to wear socks to bed OR having to dress in layers during the day OR decreased sweating OR slow to heat up with exercise)?** ____ × 2 = _____
3. ***DOUBLE SCORE* Problems with RATE of body processes (decreased reaction time OR slowed reflexes OR sluggish bowel/ constipation OR sluggish liver/ high cholesterol)?** ____ × 2 = _____

4. ***DOUBLE SCORE* Problems with ENERGY (severe fatigue OR utterly exhausted by end of day OR times during day when energy drops out completely, feeling like the plug is pulled on your energy)? ____ × 2 = ____**

5. Problems with MOOD (depression OR negative thinking OR less than full improvement taking antidepressants)? ____

6. Problems with SKIN (adult acne OR eczema OR very dry skin OR puffiness/bags around the eyes)? ____

7. Problems with HAIR (very dry like straw OR brittle OR easily breaking OR easily falling out OR loss of outer eyebrows)? ____

8. Problems with NAILS (brittle OR thin OR cracked OR peeling)? ____

9. Problems with THROAT or NECK (hoarseness for no reason OR difficulty swallowing OR easily choking OR thick tongue, frequently bitten OR intolerance to clothing/jewelry snug around neck)? ____

10. Exercise does not feel good OR muscle mass/strength does not improve with exercise? ____

Low-Thyroid Point Score Total = ____(maximum = 42)

Extra-Point Questions

Answer below if you or any of your relatives have ever been diagnosed with a low or high thyroid problem in the past, or with diabetes, rheumatoid arthritis, migraine headache, or any other autoimmune illness, like lupus, sarcoidosis, scleroderma, Sjogren's, myasthenia gravis, multiple sclerosis, Crohn's disease, ulcerative colitis, thrombocytopenia?

- If you've been diagnosed with *any*, add an extra 5 points ____
- Give a *total* of 5 more points if *any* relatives were ever diagnosed ____
- Total Extra Points ____(maximum = 10)
  Low-Thyroid Point Score Total ____ + Total Extra Points ____ = ____ (maximum = 52)

B. Could You Be HIGH Thyroid? Do You Have the Following?

1. *DOUBLE SCORE* Bulging eyes OR "Staring gaze" OR people commenting that you're looking at them too intently? ___ × 2 = _____

2. *DOUBLE SCORE* Excessively fast heart rate OR runs of skipped beats OR bothersome palpitations OR shaking of fingers or hands (tremor)? ___ × 2 = _____

3. *DOUBLE SCORE* Swelling OR tenderness of thyroid gland (goiter)? ___ × 2 = _____

4. *DOUBLE SCORE* Panic attacks or breathlessness for no reason OR unusual irritability OR hyped-up behavior change without clear cause OR general anxiety or nervousness for no apparent reason? ___ × 2 = _____

5. Feeling hot much of the time OR intolerant to heat OR sweating more than others OR pronounced warm moist skin? _____

6. Tremendous energy OR hardly needing sleep OR difficulty staying asleep? _____

7. Unusual or rapid weight loss, especially if not on a diet? _____

8. Constantly feeling like you've had too much coffee? _____

9. Loose stools, fast bowels, OR sense of metabolism "revved up"? _____

10. Light periods OR skipping periods (neither related to menopause)? _____

High-Thyroid Point Score Total = _____ (maximum = 42)

Extra-Point Questions

Answer below if you or any of your relatives have ever been diagnosed with a high thyroid problem in the past, or with diabetes or rheumatoid arthritis?

- If you've been diagnosed with *any*, add an extra 5 points ____
- Give a *total* of 5 more points if *any* relatives were ever diagnosed ____
- Total Extra Points: ____ (maximum = 10)
  High-Thyroid Point Score Total ____ + Total Extra Points = ____
  (maximum = 52)

ADRENAL GLAND EVALUATIONS

C. Could you Be LOW Adrenal? Do You Have the Following?

1. ***DOUBLE SCORE*** Easily frazzled OR flying off the handle frequently OR startling easily OR low tolerance for loud noises? ___ × 2 = _____

2. ***DOUBLE SCORE*** Poor resistance to respiratory infections OR asthma OR longer than normal recovery time from routine illness OR difficulty recuperating from unusual stress such as jet lag? Being "thrown for a loop" by small things ("the least thing just flattens me")? ___ × 2 = _____

3. ***DOUBLE SCORE*** Dizziness upon standing up OR low blood pressure OR fainting? ___ × 2 = _____

4. ***DOUBLE SCORE*** Low stamina for stress OR caving in easily OR preferring to avoid any confrontations? ___ × 2 = _____

5. Sweating or wetness of the hands when nervous? _____

6. Sense of always being stressed out OR feeling better right away when stress is resolved? _____

7. Excessive sensitivity to chemicals OR increased allergies OR low tolerance for alcohol, caffeine, other drugs, or strong odors? _____

8. Unusual fatigue, especially in the morning with more energy after meals and later as day progresses OR having better energy at night, when others are winding down (night owl)? _____

9. Salt cravings (especially liking or needing salty foods) OR lack of thirst OR markedly low blood sugar/hypoglycemia (can't skip a meal, needing snacks just to function, low fasting blood sugar on testing)? _____

10. "Tired but wired" feeling OR low reserve (little spare *oomph* to meet a challenge)? _____

Low Adrenal Point Score Total = _____ (maximum = 42)

Extra-Point Questions

Answer below if you or any of your relatives have ever been diagnosed with a low adrenal problem in the past.

- If you've been diagnosed, add an extra 5 points ____
- Give a *total* of 5 more points if *any* relatives were ever diagnosed ____

- Total Extra Points ____ (maximum = 10)
  Low Adrenal Point Score Total ____ + Total Extra Points ____ = ____ (maximum = 52)

D. Could You Be HIGH Adrenal? Do You Have the Following?

1. *DOUBLE SCORE* **Normal thinking that becomes easily confused and frazzled when rushed or under pressure?** ____ × 2 = ____
2. *DOUBLE SCORE* **Swelling/water retention of fingers OR ankles OR limbs OR face?** ____ × 2 = ____
3. *DOUBLE SCORE* **Heart palpitations OR high blood pressure?** ____ × 2 = ____
4. *DOUBLE SCORE* **Unhealthy thinning skin (easily injured or bruised) OR excessively oily skin?** ____ × 2 = ____
5. Increase in facial or body hair? ____
6. Sleep problems (staying awake much of the night)? ____
7. Elevated triglycerides? ____
8. Sugar cravings OR blood sugar imbalance? ____
9. Muscle weakness OR decreased muscle mass OR restless legs (muscle twitching at night)? ____
10. Generalized ongoing excessive tension all day long OR constant low-grade headache for days on end? ____

High Adrenal Point Score Total = ____ (maximum = 42)

Extra-Point Questions

Answer below if you or any of your relatives have ever been diagnosed with a high adrenal problem in the past.

- If you've been diagnosed, add an extra 5 points ____
- Give a *total* of 5 more points if *any* relatives were ever diagnosed ____
- Total extra points ____ (maximum = 10)

High Adrenal Point Score Total ____ + Total Extra Points ____ = _____ (maximum − 52)

WOMEN'S SEX-GLAND EVALUATIONS

E. Women, Could You Be LOW Estrogen?
Do You Have the Following?

1. *DOUBLE SCORE* **Foggy thinking OR inability to think clearly through a dilemma?** ___ × 2 = _____
2. *DOUBLE SCORE* **Hot flashes during the day OR excessive sweating at night?** ___ × 2 = _____
3. *DOUBLE SCORE* **Feeling tearful, often at slightest provocation? OR unable to cope comfortably?** ___ × 2 = _____
4. *DOUBLE SCORE* **If menstruating, early period days are your most difficult time of month?** ___ × 2 = _____
5. Sleep disturbance (either inability to fall asleep or to stay asleep)? _____
6. Memory lapses OR times when your mind goes blank OR you lose your train of thought? _____
7. Frequent headaches, either at temples or involving entire head? _____
8. Vaginal dryness (at times irritating OR making sexual contact less comfortable)? _____
9. Incontinence (inability to hold urine without leakage)? _____
10. Light and/or irregular periods, at times scanty, sometimes heavy. _____

Low Estrogen Point Score Total = _____ (maximum − 42)

Extra-Point Questions
Answer below if you or any of your relatives have ever been diagnosed with low estrogen in the past.

- If you've been diagnosed, add an extra 5 points ____
- Give a *total* of 5 more points if *any* relatives were ever diagnosed ____

- Total Extra Points ____ (maximum = 10)
  Low Estrogen Point Score Total ____ + Total Extra Points ____ =
  ____ (maximum = 52)

F. Women, Could You Be HIGH Estrogen (or Have a Progesterone Deficiency)? Do You Have the Following?

1. *DOUBLE SCORE* Exceptionally fine, smooth, "glowing" skin, hardly needing creams or any extra care? ___ × 2 = ____
2. *DOUBLE SCORE* Heavy bleeding OR uterine fibroids OR endometriosis OR extremely uncomfortable uterine symptoms? ___ × 2 = ____
3. *DOUBLE SCORE* Tender breasts, at times a sense of being bruised, or of excess fullness? ___ × 2 = ____
4. *DOUBLE SCORE* PMS time is or has been the most difficult time of month? ___ × 2 = ____
5. Fibrocystic breasts, with many little lumps that can be felt easily, OR diagnosed as chronic cystic mastitis? _____
6. Cystic ovaries, upon examination or scan, with or without abdominal discomfort? _____
7. Weight gain around the middle? _____
8. High triglycerides upon blood testing? _____
9. Anxiousness, nervousness, irritability, or foggy thinking? _____
10. Water retention, making ankles, legs, fingers, or face swollen? _____

High Estrogen Point Score Total = _____ (maximum = 42)

Extra-Point Questions
Answer below if you or any of your relatives have ever been diagnosed with high estrogen or low progesterone in the past.

- If you've been diagnosed, add an extra 5 points ____

- Give a *total* of 5 more points if *any* relatives were ever diagnosed
  ____

- Total Extra Points ____ (maximum = 10)
  High Estrogen Point Score Total ____ + Total Extra Points ____ =
  ____ (maximum = 52)

MEN'S SEX-GLAND EVALUATIONS

G. Men, Could You Be LOW Testosterone? Do You Have the Following?

1. **DOUBLE SCORE** Decreased mental ability OR decreased memory OR noticeable foggy thinking? ___ × 2 = ____
2. **DOUBLE SCORE** Decreased erection or sexual performance OR decreased sex drive? ___ × 2 = ____
3. **DOUBLE SCORE** A noticeable decrease in muscle mass? ___ × 2 = ____
4. **DOUBLE SCORE** Apathy, not caring much what happens, low motivation for life? ___ × 2 = ____
5. Slowed urine stream (decreased urine flow)? ____
6. Increased urinary urges, feeling of pressure, discomfort, or leakage (prostate problems)? ____
7. Feeling of being "burnt out"? ____
8. Decreased stamina for exercise or sexual activity? ____
9. Thinning skin, easy to bruise or scratch? ____
10. Joint stiffness OR aches and pains (neither related to arthritis)? ____

Low Testosterone Point Score Total = ____ (maximum = 42)

Extra-Point Questions

Answer below if you or any of your relatives have ever been diagnosed with low testosterone in the past.

- If you've been diagnosed, add an extra 5 points ____
- Give a *total* of 5 more points if *any* relatives were ever diagnosed ____
- Total Extra Points ____ (maximum = 10)
  Low Testosterone Point Score Total ___ + Total Extra Points ___ = ____ (maximum = 52)

H. Men, Could You Be HIGH Testosterone? Do You Have the Following?

1. *DOUBLE SCORE* **Constant pressured feeling OR almost constant irritability OR increased anxiousness for little reason?** ___ × 2 = ____
2. *DOUBLE SCORE* **Increased aggressive behavior OR excessive, near-violent responses to provocation, with little interest in conciliation?** ___ × 2 = ____
3. *DOUBLE SCORE* **Excessive body and/or facial hair (not scalp)?** ___ × 2 = ____
4. *DOUBLE SCORE* **Foggy thinking (unable to focus or think clearly)?** ___ × 2 = ____
5. Adult acne OR excessively oily skin? ____
6. Increase in loss of scalp hair? ____
7. Elevated blood lipids, especially triglycerides? ____
8. Increased headaches compared with past, pressure/pain in head? ____
9. High blood pressure? ____
10. Sleep disturbance (either unable to fall asleep or to stay asleep)? ____

High Testosterone Point Score Total = _____ (maximum = 42)

Extra-Point Questions

Answer below if you or any of your relatives have ever been diagnosed with high testosterone in the past.

- If you've been diagnosed, add an extra 5 points ____
- Give a *total* of 5 more points if *any* relatives were ever diagnosed ____
- Total Extra Points ____ (maximum = 10)
  High Testosterone Point Score Total ___ + Total Extra Points___ = ____ (maximum = 52)

SCORING AND INTERPRETING YOUR EVALUATIONS

- By now you have a Point Score Total for each of six evaluations above that pertain to your sex.
- *To determine your endo-type*, find the one evaluation out of the six with the highest total points. Whether it is low adrenal or high testosterone, this is your evaluation with the highest point score.
- If you had the most points on a thyroid evaluation, you are a **physical** endo-type. If you had the most points on a sex-hormone evaluation, you are a **mental** endo-type. If you had the most points in an adrenal evaluation, you are an **emotional** endo-type.

Keep in mind that it is only an *apparent* endo-type, until the results of your home testing are in. Because of wide differences in people's subjective sense regarding self-evaluations, there is no scale of mild, moderate, or severe in expressing your apparent endo-type.

We know that symptoms can overlap, and occasionally a person will appear to have two or all three glands as causing major health disruption. For these reasons, the home testing can provide greater definition and direction regarding which gland to address first.

For some people, your apparent endo-type will be all you need in order to begin making good corrections. Many find dramatic relief from long-term symptoms by simply rebalancing their self-evaluation–derived endo-type, which then often helps to stabilize the other glands in the body.

For example, if you are an apparent **emotional** endo-type, this may be all the information you need to greatly improve your health status. Based on this simple bit of information, you can now go directly to the adrenal rebalancing chapter (chapter 8) to initiate over-the-counter improvements in your adrenal status.

Remember Meredith, the fuzzy-thinking menopausal woman from chapter 1? Most of her *yes* answers were from the estrogen self-evaluations above. She was a **mental** endo-type with cognitive symptoms from her sex hormone imbalance.

Even though you now have an apparent endo-type, we strongly suggest that you confirm this finding by means of some simple home tests described in our next chapter. These tests can help transform an *apparent* endo-type (derived by symptoms) into an *actual* endo-type (derived by physical test results). Though this takes a bit more time and money, it is a valuable part of a proper assessment of your endocrine chemistry, and will prove very helpful in providing baseline scores that can be used in the future for rebalancing efforts.

The information available through self-evaluation questions, no matter how detailed and well scored, is just presumptive. In our experience, the most revealing result is obtained from the combination of carefully selected testing in addition to the above self-evaluations.

If you do not have the time, energy, or finances to use our suggested lab tests to *confirm* your actual endo-type, as we have said you may elect to use your apparent endo-type to guide you and your practitioner in natural, "over-the-counter" rebalancing efforts. These are explained in the individual chapters that follow. (Always do lab testing before being started on any "prescription" rebalancing medicine.) If your medical doctor does not seem to know how to help you with these natural remedies, you may need to seek a licensed naturopathic physician, knowledgeable and well-trained chiropractor, physician assistant or nurse practitioner to work with you on the fine-tuning aspects required.

Later, you might again use these same chapter 3 self-evaluations to determine if your main apparent endo-type problem has been handled, and if a different gland now needs further help.

Are you curious about how these evaluations turned out for our other two ladies, Phoebe and Emily? Each was a clear example of one of the three main endo-types. Stay tuned as we follow these women through their respective programs, helping you see more about how to improve your own gland function.

CONCEPT SUMMARY

1. Even with normal blood tests, you could easily be too high or too low in thyroid, adrenal, or sex hormones.
2. Symptoms (if analyzed carefully) are a useful way to evaluate which glands are functioning too high or too low.
3. Knowing your endo-type will help you determine which hormone needs rebalancing first in order for you to be less fat, fuzzy, or frazzled.
4. In addition, if there is more than one imbalance, your endo-type will help you to ascertain the order in which you can best approach your multigland challenge.

ACTION SUMMARY

❑ Complete the six evaluations as appropriate (above).
❑ Determine your apparent endo-type from these results.
❑ Learn all you can about your main gland challenge.
❑ Prepare for using home-testing to confirm your endo-type.

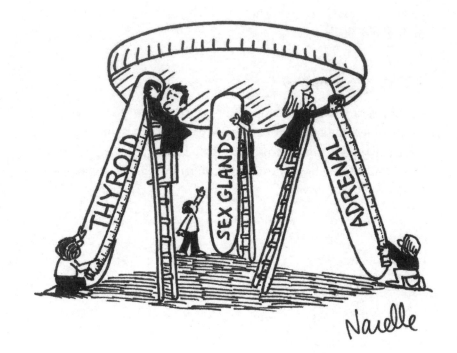

CHAPTER 4

DAY 4 OF YOUR JUMP START
CONFIRM YOUR ENDO-TYPE WITH SIMPLE HOME TESTS

Seek and ye shall find.

—Matthew 7:7

As you know from the previous chapter, Phoebe was suspected of having a low-thyroid problem, based on her self-evaluation responses. She confirmed that apparent endo-type with actual testing, as you'll learn about in this chapter. Her experience underscores the added benefit of home testing for tissue levels of hormones rather than relying strictly on blood tests, which evaluate hormone levels only in the bloodstream.

It is convenient, of course, for the lab tech in your doctor's office to stick a needle into a vein to get an idea of the specific levels of hormone in the body. It's even more convenient, less time intensive, and less invasive to take a sample of saliva at home. It's well worth seeing the level of hormone in your actual tissues.

In Phoebe's case, the level of thyroid hormone on her home test revealed a deficiency that the regular lab tests had missed. This confirmed her apparent endo-type, information that led her to seek out a much more successful treatment program.

Of all the land mines awaiting those seeking satisfactory medical solutions, few are as frustrating as testing for chronic medical complaints. In our view, inadequate testing leads to poor diagnosis, which leads to inappropriate treatment, which leads to people like yourself taking pharmaceuticals that may further cloud the picture, without fixing the cause of your problems. Conversely, appropriate testing can lead to greater efficiency and accuracy in diagnosis, therefore optimal treatment, which means you can get better quickly and get on with the life you love.

Many of you have already discovered that the majority of doctors rely almost exclusively on standard blood tests, using standard normal ranges to diagnose. Unfortunately, these tests—in addition to being costly and time consuming to perform—are surprisingly inaccurate. The new testing described in this chapter is easier to perform, less expensive, and yields more accurate results. On this fourth day, your job is simply to initiate the process of obtaining your test kit.

WHY DO TESTING AT ALL?

While a well-designed self-evaluation questionnaire is indeed useful, particularly for those who cannot do additional testing, we highly recommend saliva tests interpreted by a well-trained practitioner whenever possible. We recognize that many people have limited funding and time, yet we hope that you will corroborate your self-evaluations with simple home testing.

Faulty Self-Perception

Why not just use the questionnaires? The mind can be deceiving. Many of us have an idea about what could be our greatest strength or weakness. Sometimes, however, our own self-perception is not fully accurate. Our view of ourselves is colored by our past experiences, our wishes, our hopes, and our fears. Faulty self-perception can cloud our assessment of what might be going on in our own unique situation.

We may not be able to access adequate information to enable us to accurately evaluate what is going on in our bodies. At times our minds may negatively influence our health, such as occurs when a relative has had terrible experiences with certain conditions, and we live in fear that we may similarly be prone to those conditions.

Symptoms Overlap

Symptoms can overlap. One of the difficulties in determining your accurate hormonal profile is that many of the hormonal imbalances resemble each other in one symptom or another. For instance, a person with low thyroid can have headaches, a person with low adrenal can have headaches, and a person with low estrogen can have headaches.

With these three glands, some symptoms of one are similar to the symptoms of another. Therefore, a symptom checklist is not going to be as reliable for this situation as combining your symptom questionnaire with objective test data.

The Value of Obtaining Baseline Measurements

We highly recommend that before you embark upon any treatment program for thyroid, adrenal, or sex hormones, you obtain a comprehensive evaluation of all three of these major glands (not just the one that seems to be the presenting symptom). This can best occur using, whenever possible, a well-chosen, open-minded practitioner who has studied the interrelationships among these glands.

A baseline measurement, while not always a total reflection of your original hormone status, can allow you and your practitioners to have an idea of where you *were* before starting any new therapies.

If you have not received any hormonal correction, then your baseline testing will be accurate for that time period in your life. If you have already been taking thyroid, adrenal, or sex hormones, some labs suggest stopping their use and waiting for several months prior to testing. (Most people do not wish to do this simply to obtain an accurate baseline measurement.) For those who do choose this route, we suggest you work very carefully to make these changes, slowly cutting down in accordance with your provider's suggestions. For the majority who will not be stopping their present program, it still would be advised to measure where you are today with all three glands before proceeding further. Then, as time passes, you will have a reference point with which to compare your changing status.

WHAT'S WRONG WITH STANDARD BLOOD TESTING FOR THYROID, ADRENAL, OR SEX GLANDS?

For thousands of people we have consulted with and treated in the United States, Canada, Europe, and elsewhere, the standard testing protocols frequently have led to frustration. It can be difficult to figure out which tests to perform, in what order, how to avoid spending more time and money than is necessary on tests and—critically important—how to best interpret their results.

The Problem with Standard Testing

Many doctors, to be quite honest, don't know about the various additional, more sophisticated thyroid, adrenal, or sex-hormone tests. Change in the realm of Western medicine happens very slowly, unless there is dramatic and compelling research that immediately calls forth a clear, undisputed response. However, there are many thousands of alternative practitioners all across the country who have specialized training in this type of care.

For example, standard procedure to test for thyroid is to do just a TSH (thyroid stimulating hormone) test or in some cases, the thyroid panel, which is TSH with a Free T4. This is not really much of a panel in that there is no accurate testing for T3, which is the true *active* thyroid hormone. Also the Free T4 is a test that is commonly "normal" even when the patient is abnormal. In addition, the standard panel neglects to measure thyroid antibodies, a major marker for the cause of almost all high- and low-thyroid conditions.

In our experience, time, money, and anguish can be saved simply by performing the right tests at the beginning. Not only would health-care consumers save money, but the industry would also save perhaps many billions of dollars annually, rather than allow conditions to worsen beyond repair.

The "Range of Normal" Problem

We have already mentioned that most standardized testing has a huge range of normal, with only the most extreme results considered abnormal. Current blood testing for hormones has ranges of normal that are *way* too broad to be useful to the average person as the basis for reliable intervention. By far the most common complaint we hear from our patients is that they test in the low normal range, so they are denied treatment that could really help them.

We personally consider this problem of denial of treatment to be as serious as overtreating, when patients are given too much medicine, or put through surgeries that their bodily systems clearly can't tolerate. In our view, and that of other like-minded practitioners, this could be construed as a crime of omission, causing patients to feel worse for extended periods of time when they could easily have been helped.

The "Test Deficit" Problem

In addition to the "range of normal" problem, there is another difficulty. Blood tests are measuring the hormone level in the bloodstream. Hormones don't perform in the bloodstream. They act on the tissue level at their target sites. For complex reasons, the amount in the bloodstream does not always reflect the amount that exists at the site where the hormone will be needed. Far better is to have a testing method that actually measures the amount of hormone at the tissue level.

Some blood tests are excellent, such as a red blood count revealing anemia, a white blood count revealing infection, or a liver function test revealing hepatitis. On the other hand, standard blood tests for adrenal, thyroid, and sex hormones are very overrated, because of the blood level–tissue level dilemma.

In addition to testing for diagnostic purposes, there is the issue of using tests to optimize one's treatment. With more than 20 million people already being treated for low thyroid, it is exceedingly important to be able to determine accurately if that treatment is adequate or if it requires further adjustment.

While standard thyroid testing is often inadequate for the task of diagnosis (except in the most severe cases), we have found it even less helpful for monitoring the course of therapy. Many people, after starting the right kind of medicine, finally experience a blessed reduction in symptoms that have plagued them for years. Within weeks or months, however, their doctors insist on reducing the dose to the point where they become symptomatic again, based solely on what the blood tests show.

The patient might be feeling well for the first time in years, but the doctor instead opts for "treating the test," following standard protocol as if it was gospel. It's not.

Please realize that we are *not* suggesting that you forgo any blood testing, or that you refuse to consider having blood testing first. What we are saying is that if you are having mild health concerns, for which your own physician does not recommend further evaluation, or if your blood tests have come back normal and you're still not feeling that well, you might need to take greater charge of your own health process. Saliva testing can be an excellent beginning step to help you to pinpoint and correct subtle disorders, and they are relatively easy to use.

What We've Learned from Our Patients

When we wrote our most recent health book, *Thyroid Power*, we spent a great deal of time and energy explaining to the public about standard blood testing at regular local labs. We went into great detail about each thyroid test, what it measured, how it was used, and how to interpret results. However, after the publication of this book, we were deluged with feedback from health consumers who were righteously disgruntled with the process of standard blood testing. Many said their physicians refused to test them, based on the doctor's belief that it was not necessary and would not reveal anything helpful. Others said their doctors agreed to order testing, but then ran only one basic test. If it fell anywhere within the normal range, their doctor did not consider it important to consider whether it was almost high, or near the line indicating too low. Worse, even when the health consumers knew exactly what to ask for and why, their doctors often seemed unwilling to listen to input from them as patients.

The reality has been, sadly, that across the country, many health consumers have been unable to find physicians who will work with them to get to the bottom of their subtle hormone imbalance. Doctors are so burdened with more severe illnesses that they don't have time to adequately help someone who has mild or sometimes even moderate symptoms, as long as they can still function somewhat in the world. It may not matter that the symptoms are reducing your life force by 50 percent or more; as long as you are mobile and somewhat functional, you are not considered a sick person in need of lab testing beyond the very basic standard tests.

Rather than spend time and money on further testing, doctors readily prescribe antidepressants or tell people to eat better and to get more exercise, without educating them more fully about what these suggestions actually mean. Frequently, if there is any supportive education, it is provided by nurses who are moving more in the direction of patient education and advocacy. What we have found is that resorting to medical doctors alone is not sufficient to help those with subtle endocrine imbalance to feel better. Creative measures are clearly warranted to fill in the gaps that are allowing millions like you to fall through them.

Fortunately, helpful technology has now been developed that improves these tests. Though not entirely perfect, it is a major step forward in assessment of hormones in people with milder abnormalities, such as might make them fat, fuzzy, or frazzled. Yet, as with most changes in medicine, professionals are slow to adopt new tools. It can take many years before sensitive new testing methodology makes its way into mainstream medicine; you may not want to wait for years to receive testing that has the potential to unmask your true problems

What's Right with the New Home Tests?

A growing body of scientific literature confirms the validity of testing saliva for hormone levels (See the "Alternative Laboratories: How to Obtain Your Home Tests" section in Appendices for Web sites listing research studies.) The studies often compare levels found in saliva with those from blood testing. The comparisons have been, in general, quite positive. In considering what's right with the saliva and certain other newer tests, the answer would be that these tests are much more *accessible*, and also much more representative of a person's actual hormone status.

Accessibility

There are several reasons why people prefer using the newer testing.

Difficulty in Getting to Labs Regularly

The saliva tests permit you to perform testing in the comfort of your own home whenever you would like. You don't have to go anywhere, and you can do them on your own schedule. After collecting specimens, you simply mail the tubes to the lab in packaging provided.

Costs

Saliva testing is much less expensive than blood tests. You can generally obtain results for a whole panel of saliva tests for what it would cost you to have one single blood test. Insurance companies are beginning to provide coverage for saliva testing, and this trend will grow with greater pressure exerted from conscious consumers.

Provides More Control over Your Testing

With the home saliva tests, you get to participate in the decision about which tests are ordered. You are the one who mails off the kit, and therefore have the final say about exactly which tests are run. Most of the laboratories providing saliva testing have done extensive research on their tests, and then share this information on their Web sites. (See Lab info in Appendices.)

Specificity

Keep in mind that when hormones are released into the bloodstream, it is their purpose to go into various tissues where they have their target action. Any of the body's tissues might be fair game for assessing the amount of hormone originally in the blood that has now reached the tissue level. Saliva happens to be a very convenient substance to measure.

When you measure a hormone in *saliva*, you are measuring the actual "bioavailable" level. Hormones in the *blood* are generally tightly bound to plasma proteins. Only a tiny fraction of what is in the blood actually becomes free to enter tissues.

Saliva testing measures this free fraction (the amount of hormone that is not bound to blood proteins and is therefore free to perform in tissues). Although it has recently become possible to measure some free hormones in the blood, it is much less expensive and more accurate to measure the free fraction in saliva. It is also less invasive, less traumatic, and less time consuming.

The methods we discuss here are by no means exhaustive of what may be available. We are sharing some of the most meaningful, affordable, and helpful testing methods so you and your practitioners can begin to think more expansively, to find what works for you in monitoring your ongoing health needs.

Accuracy

In one early study, Drs. Aardal and Holm compared blood and saliva samples in 197 people. Their results demonstrated that saliva testing is superior to blood testing, since it measures free-fraction, which is the level of hormone not bound to blood proteins. (Aardal E., Holm A. C. "Cortisol in saliva-reference ranges and relation to cortisol in serum." *Eur J Clin Chem Clin Biochem* 1995; 33:927–932; also see www.salivatest.com.)

In another early study, researchers compared blood and saliva samples for adrenal hormone levels, both before and after stimulating the adrenal gland. Results showed that in almost every instance, the saliva test was similar to blood testing, validating saliva test accuracy. (Aardal-Eriksson E., Karlberg B. E., Holm A. C. "Salivary cortisol and alternative to serum cortisol determinations in dynamic function tests." *Clin Chem Lab Med* 1998; 36:215–222.)

Current hormone research published in a major medical journal compared saliva and blood testosterone levels in thirty-seven men and nine women. The results showed that saliva tesing was as accurate as blood testing, and provides a less costly, less invasive method. (Khan-Dawood F. S., Choe J. K., Dawood M. Y. "Salivary and plasma bound and "free" testosterone in men and women." *Am J Obstet Gynecol* 1984; 148:441–445.)

In addition, saliva testing is the more accurate way to measure bioavailable levels of hormones delivered topically through the skin. Since many of the recommendations in this book involve using transdermal creams, we believe saliva testing to be the most appropriate monitoring method.

THE NEW TESTS: HOW, WHEN, AND WHERE

We recommend that you evaluate your thyroid hormones, your sex-gland hormones and adrenal hormones, all at one time, on the same day. This will provide accurate baseline against which future testing can be compared. It will also serve to validate the apparent endo-type obtained from your questionnaire answers.

Here are the basic tests:

Thyroid Panel (TSH, Free T4, Free T3, microsomal antibody)
Menstruating Woman: Sex-Hormone Panel (estrogen, progesterone, testosterone)
Menopausal Woman: Sex-Hormone Panel (estrogen, progesterone, testosterone)
Men: Sex-Hormone Panel (testosterone, estrogen, progesterone)
Adrenal Stress Panel (four samples for cortisol and DHEA)

Each of these panels is explained more fully in this chapter in the section below pertaining to that specific endo-type.

Recommended Labs

We have listed a number of the very best labs in the United States in our Appendices on page 251. If you call them on their toll-free lines, each of them would be happy to discuss the tests they offer, their efficacy, as well as how to perform them.

Specifically, Diagnos-Techs Lab in Kent, Washington (www .diagnostechs.com) will check for thyroid using the new saliva method of home testing. They run adrenal and sex-hormone determinations by saliva, as well.

We also especially recommend ZRT Labs in Beaverton, Oregon (www.salivatest.com), BioHealth in Santa Monica, California (www .biohealthinfo.com), and Great Smokies Lab in Asheville, North Carolina (www.gsdl.com).

The Appendices in the back of the book will provide you and your practitioners with more information about competent labs from which you may obtain a test kit. While you can sometimes obtain these kits on your own and have results sent directly to you, we highly recommend that you also work with a knowledgeable practitioner to help you interpret your test results. This can be an open-minded MD, chiropractor, naturopath, osteopathic doctor, acupuncturist, nutritionist, nurse practitioner or physician assistant.

If you are unable to find a practitioner in your area, it might be possible to have the test ordered or receive help with interpretation via membership in an organization called the Canary Club. (For details, see www.canaryclub.org)

Often the lab can also refer you to doctors practicing in the vicinity who use their lab. Also in our Appendices' "For More Information" section is a list of organizations whose professional members generally order tests from these laboratories for their patients.

Specific Suggestions for Testing

Each lab will have its own set of instructions that will explain collection procedure in great detail included in the collection kit. It can be mailed directly to you or to your cooperating provider, some of whom have such kits in their offices already. Results from these labs can also be sent to both you and your practitioner. For now, here are the basic ideas.

Sex-Gland Evaluation

You may want to do the standard minimum saliva panel. At most labs, this is an estradiol, a progesterone, and a testosterone level. Men and menopausal women can do this one saliva sample testing on any day of any month.

Women who are menstruating should do the test on day nineteen or twenty of their cycle when possible. (Day one is the day you start to bleed.)

Adrenal Testing

There is one test generally called Adrenal Profile or Adrenal Stress Index (ASI). This involves one saliva sample collected in the morning before breakfast, another sample collected around noon (before lunch), another around 4 p.m. (before dinner), and another around 10 p.m. (before bed). Some labs offer this test as a two-sample collection. We suggest that you complete a four-sample test when possible.

Thus you have four separate samples collected several hours apart, between meals, to get your daily range of cortisol and DHEA levels. Normally cortisol is high in the morning, lower at lunch, still lower later in the day, and lowest at bedtime. Comparing yourself to the normal curve (supplied by the lab in your kit) can be quite revealing.

Testing for Thyroid Hormone

This test can be done with saliva at one particular lab (Diagnos-Techs Lab in Kent, Washington). Generally it has been more challenging to do thyroid testing by saliva, so this particular lab has for years been running blood samples parallel to saliva samples at no extra charge while improving its saliva technology for thyroid. The correlation has been good, with frequent occasions where saliva determination has been superior.

The ZRT Lab in Beaverton, Oregon, tests for thyroid levels via blood-spot testing. This involves a fairly painless finger prick, then putting a few drops of blood on a small piece of filter paper. This then gets mailed to the lab for analysis. Blood-spot testing uses gas chromatography to analyze dried specimens. It is more accurate than blood analysis, especially for the gold-standard TSH determinations. This is because pituitary hormones like TSH degrade rapidly when kept as a liquid in blood tubes, waiting to be analyzed. (The other alternative labs mentioned generally provide thyroid testing by regular blood draw at a local lab's draw station, and including that Blood tube with the Saliva kit that is mailed to the alternative lab with your saliva samples.)

In addition, thyroid determination can be done via measurement of basal temperature. A majority of people who show low body temperatures are low thyroid. This is a time-tested and helpful beginning step to determining if thyroid is involved in your situation.

To do this basal temperature determination, it is recommended that you obtain a basal (nondigital, nonmercury) thermometer if you can find it. Take your temperature for ten minutes *before* getting out of bed in the early morning. Measure your temperature by placing the thermometer in your armpit, with your arm comfortably at your side.

At the end of ten minutes, remove thermometer, read and record your reading. (The reason the armpit is used for basal temp is that there can be mild infections in the mouth, nose, ears, or sinuses that will cause oral temperature to record as higher than overall body temperature.) Repeat this process for at least five consecutive days. Then after five to seven days of recording readings, add them up and find your average temperature reading. If it is below 97.6 degrees, you are showing signs of hypothyroidism, which slows down the body's metabolic processes.

Men and postmenopausal women can do this test at any time during the month. Menstruating women should do this test starting on the third day of their cycle (with day one being the first day of bleeding).

HOW TO INTERPRET THE TESTS AND NEXT STEPS

On this fourth day of your jump start, you simply initiate the home testing process by ordering your test kit. Later you do the sample collection. You may mail off the kit to the lab after that. A prepaid mailing envelope is usually provided. The specimens will remain stable for many days.

Once mailed, samples will be evaluated at the chosen laboratories, and the results sent back either to you or your health practitioner or both. The results are presented in a format that is easy for you and your practitioner to understand. The test results contain explanatory text along with the raw data, along with graphs to show how your results compare to what is considered normal.

Basically, what you will receive back from the labs are your levels of each of the three different glands' functional output. Your results might be normal, too high, or too low. This information will help you confirm and refine your apparent endo-type, as originally assessed by the earlier questionnaires.

Having now a more objective assessment of your endo-type will allow you to proceed with very sensible and effective methods to reestablish balance. Whichever of your three main glands shows itself to be most abnormal, is the gland to start rebalancing and recharging first. If you had more than one gland out of balance, then we highly recommend you rebalance and recharge in the order of greatest severity.

In other words, if thyroid is your major abnormality, start rebalancing the thyroid first. Your task is to restore thyroid balance before moving to the other glands.

Once you have indeed established more appropriate thyroid levels, then you might proceed to rebalance the next most needy gland. You would do this only, however, after perhaps a few months' time, allowing the thyroid to rebalance fully, so you can determine by how you feel if, in fact, further attention is required. Many times the effort involved in balancing the main culprit results in improvement of the other glands, as well. This shift often makes it unnecessary to address specific rebalancing for the other glands.

If you mainly show adrenal abnormality on self-evaluation and lab testing, it would therefore be most appropriate to start with adrenal balancing. The same is true for the sex hormones, as well.

Remember, in the case of discrepancy, these tests carry more weight than the questionnaires.

Proceeding in this way will allow you the best chance for true and lasting success. We have seen thousands of people, women especially, coming in to our office, claiming that they have felt lousy for years. Many have been handed sex hormone drugs, with estrogens, as a first step. This all too common but unfortunate misstep often resulted in more years of feeling poorly. Beneath the sex-hormone challenge there is often either an adrenal or a thyroid imbalance. That more primary imbalance needed to be taken care of first.

Working with us, a great many of these hormone sufferers found their best route to recovery. Interpreting your tests and then making good use of them, is the proper place to start.

CONCEPT SUMMARY

1. Standard blood tests are costly, inconvenient, and not as accurate for your purposes as the newer cutting-edge, home test technology.
2. Saliva, blood spot, and temperature testing can actually be more accurate for this purpose than standard blood testing.
3. The home tests to include are a thyroid panel, an adrenal stress index, and a basic sex-hormone panel. These are available from a number of reputable laboratories.
4. The gland that shows the greatest abnormality upon testing is the one that should be addressed first. This will generally be the gland that showed the highest distress on the questionnaires.
5. If there is a difference between the results of questionnaires (apparent endo-type) and those of testing (actual endo-type), we recommend considering test results as more definitive.

ACTION SUMMARY

❑ In order to verify your endo-type, we recommend testing the hormonal output of each of your three main energy glands.

❑ Have a testing kit mailed to you. Use it to collect samples in the comfort and convenience of your own home. Once you have collected specimens, you simply mail the test kit back to the lab.

❑ Since details vary from lab to lab, check with your chosen lab's Web site or 800 number for specific costs, insurance coverage, and turn-around time.

❑ The determinations you seek are a Thyroid Panel (TSH, Free T4, Free T3, and Thyroid Antibody), a Sex-Hormone panel (estrogen, progesterone, testosterone), and an Adrenal Stress Panel (four samples of cortisol and DHEA).

❑ When you receive your test results, you and your practitioner can use them to ascertain if one, two, or all three of these major glands are functioning at too high or too low an output.

❑ Depending on which gland system shows most abnormal, you may now begin rebalancing and recharging that gland.

❑ If needed, any of these determinations can be further refined or corroborated with advanced blood testing. This will be discussed in the individual chapters on thyroid, adrenal, and sex-hormone balance.

❑ Details for rebalancing each of these major glands, and having them coexist in harmony with the other two, constitute the full program of this book, as presented in chapters soon to follow.

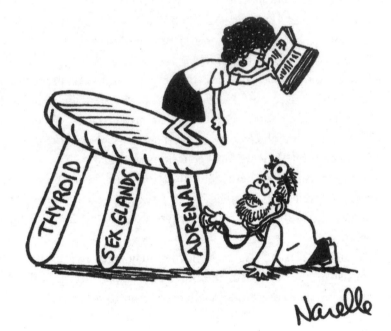

CHAPTER 5

DAY 5 OF YOUR JUMP START
SET THE STAGE FOR SUCCESS

All excesses are inimical to Nature. It is safer to proceed a little at a time, especially when changing from one regimen to another.

—Hippocrates

Emily, our young, agitated stockbroker, was still frazzled, finding little help from either the medical profession or standard over-the-counter interventions. Her efforts to get extra sleep were not of benefit. She was increasingly hostile and agitated toward friends and coworkers.

Based on her self-evaluation scores and the results of her saliva testing, it was easily determined that she was mainly an adrenal-driven endo-type. We first encouraged her to engage in more vigorous activity than stretching.

We also recommended a very strong multivitamin product with minerals to help support her glandular system more effectively. We suggested that she cease drinking regular coffee and instead begin to substitute with decaffeinated, which actually proved very helpful by reducing the dietary overstimulation of her adrenal gland. This led to an immediate reduction in her agitation without a decline in her energy, thanks to the addition of salsa dancing, something she'd long wanted to try.

The decaf was actually less bitter than the stronger regular coffee, which meant Emily was able to use less of her usual artificial sweetener.

Decreasing the caffeine and artificial sweetener along with the addition of a few basic vitamins helped the stomach problem to resolve.

Emily soon began to feel more like her old self, with less jittery behavior and better control over her nerves. Her initial jump start was beginning to pay off, increasing her interest in knowing more. Without that burning feeling in her stomach, she was actually less agitated.

GENERAL GUIDELINES FOR ALL ENDO-TYPES

How might you immediately utilize the information from chapters 1 through 4? The following start-up recommendations are applicable for everyone.

No matter which endo-type you are now, you can jump-start your health with these positive actions.

After these universal jump-start actions, we will share more personalized advice for each particular endo-type. This will include initial diet, vitamin, and exercise suggestions for thyroid, adrenal, and sex-hormone challenges respectively.

Immediate Action for All Endo-Types

- Add specific **high-quality supplements** known to be helpful for people challenged by hormonal imbalance. Keep in the forefront of your mind that for these conditions, the topic of nutrient quality is critically important. People with gland imbalance require the highest quality, lowest allergenicity of vitamins and minerals such as we list on page 257. Regular supermarkets and drug stores do not carry this level of product. You need to shop at a health food or vitamin store with a positive reputation, or find one of the better companies online. Knowing how difficult and confusing this can be, we have made suggestions in a special section of the Appendices called "Locating Your Recommended Vitamins." Please read this material carefully prior to shopping for your hormone rebalancing supplements.

- Start with a good **multivitamin and multimineral combination** supplement. Look for a high-quality item such as the multivitamin preparations listed in our "Recommended Vitamin" section, which reflect our best judgment and years of experience. For your added convenience in ordering vitamins, please see page 257 of Appendices. If you are extremely careful and knowledgeable, you might shop locally at nondiscount health or vitamin stores that have highly trained staff competent to answer your questions. If you are taking prescription pills, it is best to take any extra calcium and iron (over and above your multivitamin) twelve hours before or after taking thyroid medication.

- Add a **full-symphony antioxidant** mix once each day. One pill of a high-quality product might include (but not be limited to) vitamins A, C, E, zinc, and selenium, glutathione, N-acetylcysteine, green tea extract, milk thistle, grape seed extract, and so forth. Since the mixed antioxidants vary greatly in the choice of nutrients and their concentrations, we have not listed specific amounts. You are best advised to go with a good company that is known to do a fine job with this kind of mix. One example is the product Oxygenics from the Metagenics company; another is Oraxinal from the Xymogen company.

- Include an ample dose of **omega-3 and omega-6 fatty acids.** They are called essential fatty acids (or EFAs) because the main two categories, linoleic acid (omega-6) and linolenic acid (omega-3) cannot be made by the human body; therefore, they must be included in your diet. Make sure you get at least 500 mg of omega-3 and 250 mg of omega-6 daily. They help with attachment and active transport of fluid into the cells via maintenance and repair of the receptor sites, allowing greater utilization of thyroid hormone. Make sure that the brand you purchase has been screened or filtered for contaminants, especially mercury. It should say on the label "from farmed fish" or "tested for heavy metals", or "filtered free of environmental pollutants" (PCBs, dioxins, pesticides, and heavy metals).

- Now add 1 gram daily of an **amino acid mix.** The absolute best version of such a mix would be labeled "free-form aminos," 500 mg per pill. (Other versions are effective as well.) Take two daily with breakfast, along with all your other supplements. These are the building blocks for many of your hormones and neurotransmitters.

FIRST INTERVENTIONS FOR EACH SPECIFIC ENDO-TYPE

Depending upon your particular endo-type, specific *additional* vitamins and dietary maneuvers will help initiate a restoration of balance.

Feeling Fat: The **Physical** Endo-Type

You may feel that you don't have as much energy as you need, and could easily give up. It is very important that you conserve your energy carefully. Simple, effective ways to do this will be presented in chapter 12. Depression or lack of hope can be related to your lack of proper hormone levels. You may be dealing with excess weight because your metabolism is slowed.

Many annoying medical problems often go with this territory. Medicines frequently do not have their expected benefits, and their side effects can be unusual or excessive. Blood tests generally show that everything is in the normal range, adding to the frustration. **Physical** endo-types can feel like there is a slow ebbing of life force, with their essence becoming weaker and weaker. People often describe this experience with the words, "I feel like half my former self."

To begin to improve, you will need to get plenty of rest and sleep and to guard your energy carefully. This may mean being more selective about who you allow into your world.

Immediate Actions for the **Physical** Endo-Type

- **Diet:** The best foods for a thyroid type are items that *are high in fiber and low in calories*. For many people, this ends up being somewhat of a vegetarian diet with plenty of non-animal protein sources. If your metabolism is sluggish, you want to support your intestine as it transports the food through its length, which is helped by extra fiber (and slowed by meat and dairy). This type of high complex carbohydrate way of eating is similar to the diets of McDougall, Pritikin, and Ornish.

Also, since you may have sluggish metabolism, you would naturally want to satisfy your urge to eat with foods that have the highest bulk, crunchiness, taste appeal, visual attractiveness, but which are low in calories. This all adds up to eating more fruits, vegetables, beans, seeds, nuts, and sprouts. To help handle the autoimmune issues related to thyroid, include plenty of avocados and olives, even though they are not highly recommended by the diet specialists above.

Try to select fresh, whole, organically grown items whenever possible.

Buy in bulk from a reputable health food store, or even through co-op or Internet organic sales. Not only will you save money, but also you will end up with fewer additives and more nutrients. (We will elaborate on this type of diet lifestyle in chapter 9, but for now we suggest that you simply get started, as quickly or as slowly as suits your taste.)

- *Supplements:* The best additional beginning recommendation, if you are a **physical** endo-type, is to focus on the key metabolic minerals. Simply put, *in addition to a multiple vitamin and antioxidant,* you need

  200 micrograms (mcg) *extra* selenium
  200 mcg *extra* chromium
  400 mg *extra* magnesium

Of particular importance for the thyroid endo-type is the addition of the mineral **selenium.** *This one step is the key to many people's thyroid balance, or lack thereof.* It is a crucial cofactor in the five-prime-deiodinase enzyme, which takes one atom of iodine off the prohormone molecule of T4, thereby converting it into a molecule of T3, the active thyroid hormone.

Often the thyroid gland produces enough T4, or frequently people are taking enough T4 (Synthroid or other brands of thyroxine) but the T4 does not get converted adequately into the active compound T3. When you don't have enough T3, you are hypothyroid—regardless of how much T4 is floating around. Because selenium is sometimes in poor supply in the standard American diet, we are strongly recommending that **physical** endo-types continuously take in this additional 200 mcg per day over and above what is in your multivitamin-and-mineral combo. Your thyroid will thank you.

- *Exercise:* The **physical** endo-type is generally short on energy. You may not at first have the steam and stamina for vigorous exercise. Rebalancing will restore your lost oomph eventually, while for now you'd best start with more gentle activity. The recommended body movement for you is regular, repetitive, rhythmic activity. This includes walking and *easygoing versions* of swimming, cycling, treadmill, StairMaster, rowing, or NordicTrack.

If even the sound of these makes you feel tired, first just try some simple deep breathing to help you feel more alert. Then try a little walking, even if it's only five minutes once a day. Gradually increase to twice daily. Then increase your times to about twenty minutes, and do it at least three or four times a week.

Do not push beyond your endurance. Stay within your breath, and build tolerance gradually. If you feel tired at certain times each day, do what you can to add five or ten minutes of exercise at those slump times, (even pretending to run very gently in place, stretching before and after), allowing yourself to breathe fully and release fully.

If you are seated throughout much of your day, make a point of getting up every hour (without fail) and moving. Make small circles with your hips, rotate your wrists and shoulders, fingers and arms, and gently move the head from side to side. Breathe.

As your tolerance increases, you can add other forms of exercise, as indicated in chapter 9. More specific nutritional recommendations will be provided in chapter 6.

- *To Avoid:* One of the most crucial categories to steer clear of if you are a **physical** endo-type is the **halogen elements** fluorine, chlorine, bromine. Anything more than trace amounts of these substances can interfere with your thyroid metabolism, since they compete with the precise amount of iodine needed by your thyroid gland for production of thyroid hormone.

Unfortunately, these halogens are extremely common in the environment, as mentioned in chapter 2. Try to find nonfluoridated toothpaste in the health food store. Never breathe in or spill chlorine bleach on yourself. Be very careful when adding bromine to spas and hot tubs. Avoid anything more than the small amount of iodine that is generally contained in your multivitamin. This minimum dosage ensures that you will have an adequate amount as needed for thyroid hormone production. People living in the interior of the United States are best advised to use iodized salt, while those who live on the coasts and eat seafood may want to use noniodized salt.

> *At our recommendation, Phoebe added a strong full-symphony antioxidant combo to her vitamin regimen. Since many thyroid problems are inflammatory in nature (the most common cause of low thyroid is thyroiditis, "itis" referring to inflammation), the anti-inflammatory effect of the strong antioxidants was enormously beneficial to her, allowing her thyroid gland to secrete appropriate amounts of thyroid hormone more comfortably.*
>
> *Phoebe now experienced relief from her constipation and dry skin. She wasn't as sluggish as before, enabling her to work more comfortably on her swing shift position. There was even a sense that the hair loss was slowing. She was eager to learn about some of the more specific and powerful rebalancing tools promised in chapter 6.*

Fuzzy-Thinking: The **Mental** Endo-Type

As you likely already know, the challenges of this endo-type are often related to your ability to focus. It can affect your drive to achieve, your concentration, spark, edge, focus, determination, and clear (versus foggy) thinking, in addition to sexual challenges. You may have to work harder than others to make a coherent case that is perceived as clear communication by the busy people around you.

Daily life, not to mention navigating the medical system, requires good, focused spark. Your foggy thinking can prevent success just when you need it most. These qualities may result in immobilization, where you can't think clearly to make good decisions. You might find yourself in the position of gathering different information from a variety of providers, and then being unable to decipher the most appropriate health strategy consistent with your beliefs and values. Meditation and deep breathing can be very helpful beginning steps as you move ahead on your program.

Immediate Actions for the **Mental** Endo-Type

- **Diet:** The best diet to follow if you are the sex gland–driven **mental** endo-type is *high protein*. To counter the tendency to be scattered or unfocused, you will need a steady supply of good solid grounding food for long-term comfort. This generally means you could benefit from a higher protein intake for a more solid nutritional foundation. The most familiar popular plans for this way of eating are the Atkins diet and Sugar Busters.

Herein lies a quandary—how to get high protein without eating way too much fat? Obviously if you are eating meats, they should be the leanest cuts possible. Perhaps better than red meat would be to rotate and include liberal amounts of free-range organic chicken or turkey without the skin. Those of you who like the white meat part of the bird are fortunate, because there is less fat in light meat than in dark meat.

If you purchase canned or frozen poultry, read the label carefully and select *low-fat meats*. A label entry that says TURKEY has much more fat than one that says TURKEY MEAT. But even this will have more fat than one that says TURKEY BREAST. More and more stores are labeling the fat percentages today, so encourage your markets to label appropriately, and choose carefully.

Whether you eat red meat or poultry or both, always insist that the product you purchase is *hormone-free*. You may have to talk to the store manager, or shop at health food supermarkets when available. As consumers begin to demand this, more delicatessens and meat departments are beginning to seek out hormone-free beef, chicken, turkey, lamb, and others.

- *Supplements:* In addition to a multivitamin and an antioxidant, the number-one best supplement to further focus on if you are a **mental** endo-type is much more of one omega-3 fatty acid (in addition to the general recommendation earlier in the chapter for all endo-types).

For your good mental function, you need a high dose of this particular fatty acid. The best source of this omega-3 is fish, *especially the fish oil*. Two particular components of fish oil are the EPA and the DHA (docosahexanoic acid), and the one we are recommending more of is the first, EPA. This oil is antiinflammatory, as well as immune boosting, and mood elevating.

The way to help your focus and memory right away would be to take an additional 300 mg of fish oil, yielding approximately 1,000 IUs of DHA and 2,000 IUs of EPA. This is your daily dose of a valuable mental supplement, in addition to your general vitamin protocol. If you have already been on such a regimen for some time, and are looking for further benefit, additional recommendations for your endo-type will be found in chapter 8.

- *Exercise:* What kind of exercise is best for the **mental** endo-type? The answer in a word is *yoga.* Here we have slow stretching combined with total focus and concentration. This is a type of exercise that will sharpen that foggy mind and increase your ability to stay on target.

When properly executed, a yoga posture involves absolute devotion to one particular form over the course of one to several minutes. During this time, you are to focus on not only the desired direction of stretch, but also on the degree of stretch. You need to focus on whether you are

at that exquisite edge between yoga being interesting versus being uncomfortable, as well as focusing on your rate and depth of breathing. All
the while, you are moving toward and away from your edge, breathing
into any discomfort and releasing it through the breath. Total focus,
total awareness, total concentration, total balance.

For those unfamiliar with yoga, it is simply comprised of slow, gentle stretching to the point that it feels interesting, coupled with an awareness of how your body feels at each point of the stretch.

An example? Bend forward gently, as if to touch your toes. This is an
exercise performed throughout the world, and is also a yoga posture.
You don't even have to touch your toes. The goal is to feel the stretch,
regardless of how far into it you can get physically.

When performed with awareness, the process takes place slowly,
over a couple of minutes, gradually coming closer and closer to your full
stretch, all the while breathing very slowly, in and out, to help you concentrate fully on what you are doing. You can simply do this as slow
stretching with various parts of your body, or you could actually get involved with yoga, where the stretching posture is called an asana.

In addition to the posture or asana, you can focus your mental apparatus even further with a greater exploration of your breathing. This is
called pranayama. It is a recommended yoga activity to simply sit and
engage in a variety of well-differentiated breathing patterns. This is the
yoga of the breath, and although awareness of breathing generally ac-
companies the postures, it can also be practiced as a separate science
unto itself.

- *To Avoid:* Once again, eliminate hormones from your foods.
  These are often found in red meats and poultry unless you buy
  organic, hormone-free products. The **mental** endo-type has enough
  problems with hormones already without adding to the confusion through food intake.

Recall that a major source of estrogenic hormone is pesticides. The
mental endo-type should avoid any bug sprays, chemical insect repel-
lents, and other hormonally active pest products. It would be much better for you to deal with the pest than to have your mental apparatus

further clouded in this way! Moreover, you would ideally use natural cleaning products, such as vinegar, club soda, or specially prepared non-toxic products. (We have listed several excellent reference books in our "Further Reading" section.)

Additionally, we suggest that you avoid buying meats or cheeses that are encased in clear plastic or cling wrap. The plasticizers used in production of these filmy materials leach out into the fat, and they can become a hormone disruptor for you.

If you are taking prescription hormones already, the recommendations in this chapter are perfectly safe, and may actually help further balance your situation. In general, we recommend taking your supplements once a day, in the morning. For those taking thyroid medicine in the morning, we suggest moving any calcium and iron to bedtime.

The best general advice we were able to give Meredith, after she discontinued the oral birth control, was to carefully consider the quality of meat and poultry she was consuming. Commonly these foods can have enough hormones to tip the scale uncomfortably in someone who is already dominant in estrogen, and exquisitely sensitive to it.

Meredith had been, appropriately, eating a high-protein diet, which is encouraged for her endo-type. But it turned out that the ranchers from whom her supermarket purchased poultry used estrogenic hormones to plump up the birds. While this is a common practice, sanctioned by governmental authorities as being safe in general, it was extremely uncomfortable for Meredith in particular, contributing to her overall memory or focus problems.

When she began to seek out only hormone-free meat and poultry, she noticed a gradual improvement in her ability to concentrate and think clearly. Not only was she more focused, but her swollen breasts shrank, as well. This encouraged her to want to try some of the specific rebalancing maneuvers that were available through our clinic. We'll see more about how that went for her in chapter 7.

Frazzled: The **Emotional** Endo-Type

More than likely, you have been living in fight-or-flight mode. In dealings with daily life and with the medical system, however, this may not be helpful. You might be viewed as a "problem patient" by your health providers. Alternatively you might be considered a fearful and anxious person difficult to get along with.

You will need to work on keeping your anxiety down, and to prevent flipping back and forth in your mind, emotions, and responses. Stress-reduction activities would help enormously, even though it may seem to you that there is no time for them. In chapter 7, we will explain much more about how stress affects your life, in countless ways, and how to reclaim a more relaxed state. Then in chapter 11 we share more about activities to help you maintain a peaceful state for the long haul.

For now, however, we encourage you to start by making the following suggestions an initial component of your program.

Immediate Actions for the **Emotional** Endo-Type

- **Diet:** An adrenal-driven endo-type needs to have her biochemistry evened out. It is generally way too jagged, with peaks and valleys, outbursts and meltdowns and eruptions that would ideally be modulated to reduce these excessive swings. The popular diet plans utilizing this middle-of-the road approach are the South Beach Diet and The Zone.

Nutritionally speaking, a great leveler is **complex carbohydrate.** We therefore recommend that you drastically reduce or eliminate your intake of *simple* carbohydrates, including white-flour pasta and bakery goods, as well as breads and pizza. It also means cutting way back on any sweets. We know these are comfort foods for many people, but they come at too high a price for **emotional** endo-types. Cookies, pies, pudding, cake, candy, pastries—all taste sweet in the short run. Over the course of several hours, however, they jack your energy around in a ruthless, unforgiving manner.

Instead, try whole grains. For breakfast, consider oatmeal (without sugar) or Cream of Wheat, skipping any syrup or orange juice. For lunch, we suggest a fresh vegetable salad with a bit of protein, such as salmon or chicken. For dinner, use whole-grain brown rice with smaller amounts of meat and vegetables.

For those who feel that they need more to eat, you can augment the above intake with small amounts of sprouted breads, pastas containing whole grains, and potatoes. These complex carbohydrates burn slowly and can keep your blood sugar more even.

- *Supplements:* Initial supplement guidelines for the **emotional** endo-type include a focus on the B vitamins. Take an additional **B-complex** pill each morning with breakfast. Also add extra **pantothenic acid,** a key B vitamin for the care and feeding of the adrenal gland. We suggest that you take 500 mg over and above whatever amount might be in your general multivitamin and in your additional B-complex.

- *Exercise:* First, you need to know that it makes a huge difference whether you are high or low adrenal endo-type in terms of exercise recommendation.

  A *high-adrenal* person is often tired and wired at the same time. This is the kind of person who does well using vigorous, even competitive exercise to burn off extra adrenal hormone. While ideally you would know when you are highest and lowest in adrenal hormones, you can experiment with exercising at various times of day. Most of the time, a high adrenal person benefits from exercising first thing in the morning, when adrenal hormones are likely to be highest.
  A *low-adrenal* person feels just plain exhausted, with very low tolerance for any stress at all. This person needs much less exercise. **Emotional** endo-types often overdo it. Any amount of exercise is too much for you at this time, if it makes you feel worse while you're doing it, a couple of hours later, or especially if you're worse the day after because of the exercise

- *To Avoid:* Food additives and synthetic chemicals are extremely harmful to the sensitive adrenal glands. If you are the **emotional** endo-type, be extra vigilant to avoid anything that you can't pronounce, or that sounds like a chemical additive or preservative.

High-quality organic foods, whether prepackaged or frozen, have labels that read like a home cookbook; only foods and spices are listed. The labels of the foods you eat should look like that.

One of the most difficult chemicals for the **emotional** endo-type to deal with is found in coffee beans and cola nuts. Yes, we're talking about *caffeine*. It is essential for an adrenal-challenged person to reduce, and if possible eliminate, her caffeine intake. Even though this is a chemical that is used very commonly in societies the world over, and in different forms, it is a terrible problem for **emotional** endo-types. It overdrives the adrenal gland, as well as the central nervous system that talks to the adrenal gland. You will have a tremendous improvement in your adrenal/emotional recovery if you can manage to reduce or stay away from caffeine.

The suggestions in this chapter complete your jump start. This may end up being all you need to know for recovery of your hormone balance. Generally, however, additional balancing is needed to fully achieve your goals. In that case, you may want to make use of the full program, which follows in chapters 6, 7, or 8, depending upon your particular endo-type.

It is up to you to take charge and move your agenda ahead. This involves understanding as much as possible about your specific endo-type, and taking more personalized steps for reclaiming your health. Whenever you are ready, an additional whole chapter on each endo-type awaits you.

CONCEPT SUMMARY

1. All endo-types can jump-start their health program with the general steps that include vitamins, stress reduction, exercise, plus structured rest and rejuvenation.
2. Taking specific additional steps for your individual endo-type will further set the stage for success.
3. Understanding your own endo-typical traits helps you choose the best practitioners for your particular needs.
4. Taking charge of your health program improves your inner bio-

chemical responses, boosting immunity and your chances for success.

5. Surround yourself with positive supportive people, including your health team members.

6. Keep in mind that healing is a journey, an art, and a process. Enjoy it all, and remember to let your inner guidance direct your path!

ACTION SUMMARY

Jump Start for All Endo-Types

❑ Strong multivitamin/mineral product daily
❑ Additional high-quality antioxidant tablet daily
❑ Extra essential fatty acids daily (500 mg omega-3, 250 mg omega-6)
❑ Extra (free-form) amino acids daily (two 500 mg capsules)

Specific Jump-Start Steps for **Physical** Endo-Types

❑ *Diet:* High vegetable, high-fiber, organic foods
❑ *Supplements:* Extra minerals—selenium 200 mg, magnesium 400 mg (magnesium citrate preferred), chromium 200 mg
❑ *Exercise:* Regular, rhythmic, repetitive gentle aerobic activity

Specific Jump-Start Steps for **Mental** Endo-Types

❑ *Diet:* High protein, hormone free
❑ *Supplements:* Extra EPA, preferably from fish oil (500 mg)
❑ *Exercise:* slow, focused stretching (such as yoga)

Specific Jump-Start Steps for **Emotional** Endo-Types

❑ *Diet:* Middle-of-the-road, complex carbs
❑ *Supplements:* Extra B-complex plus additional B-5 (pantothenic)
❑ *Exercise:*
    For high adrenal—full vigorous workout
    For low adrenal—minimal lighter workout

STEP II

INTERMEDIATE REBALANCING TOOLS

INTRODUCTION TO STEP II

Now that you have a jump start on reclaiming your endo-balance, you are ready to utilize a variety of powerful tools to help adjust and fully restore your energy glands. Here you will find detailed methods using the appropriate nutritional supplementation and natural remedies to resolve the problem. Also here are the prescription medicine protocols utilized at our clinic and, generally, by physicians or other licensed providers who have been trained in the use of bioidentical and natural hormone therapies. You are encouraged to discuss these with your doctor if you feel that even stronger balancing is needed.

Remember to start slowly and progress carefully, adding one item at a time and allowing several weeks for changes to equalize. While reviewing the material for your specific endo-type, keep in mind that most of us are a mix of these three patterns, with one that is currently predominant. If your results from chapters 3 and 4 suggest that you have strong influences from other endo-types, then be sure to read all related chapters, balancing first your primary gland, then addressing others later if needed.

It is imperative that anyone who is pregnant or contemplating pregnancy work with a careful knowledgeable practitioner before adding any nutritional supplement or herbs.

Lastly, we recommend that you keep a notebook or journal to track what has worked and what hasn't. In this way, you can refer back to these notes in the future if needed, and continue to make forward progress over time.

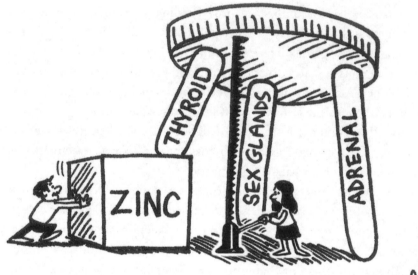

CHAPTER 6

REDUCE FAT:
BOOST A TIRED THYROID
Vitamins, Minerals, Herbs, and Prescriptions

Now is the hour that requires great help.

—Virgil

*Phoebe had begun to address her newly discovered thyroid situation with the general recommendations from chapter 5. These included a high-quality multivitamin with minerals. The additional zinc and selenium in this stronger product, along with the other items she took, seemed to be just what her thyroid needed. She was indeed a **physical** endo-type.*

The high dose, full spectrum antioxidant had already begun to work on the annoying secondary symptoms of constipation, dry skin, and hair loss. But Phoebe was still somewhat sluggish and very overweight, given that her diet was generally good.

We suggested a more specific intervention now that her apparent endo-type had been confirmed by the home tests. We recommended that Phoebe purchase an item called thyroid glandular. This is actual thyroid gland tissue of animal origin with most of the active ingredients removed, so that it can be sold at vitamin or health food stores rather than as prescription medicine.

The extra raw materials and building blocks provided by the glandular substance often have a positive effect on a sluggish thyroid system. In addition, there may be very small but still useful amounts of the active T-3 and T-4 thyroid hormones available in the over-the-counter product. Sometimes this is just enough to tip the scale in a favorable direction.

Researchers have suggested that even a tiny amount of help with thyroid hormone levels can be enough to reduce the autoimmune effect.

In addition to the glandular, we recommended that Phoebe take an herbal mix called Padma Basic to normalize and cool down her immune system. This formula, described more fully below, is actually a prescription medicine in Europe, because it is so effective, but is available over the counter here in the United States. (See Appendix 2 for more information.)

With these specific rebalancing maneuvers, Phoebe regained most of her lost energy, and she was able to lose almost a pound a week.

How could advanced medical science miss such simple, effective interventions? The answer lies in the unpredictable or erratic ways that the glands begin to malfunction. A gland is simply a factory, whose job it is to produce a hormone. The factory production can fluctuate up and down considerably before there is actual total failure. This is similar to other organs, but frequently other organs fail in a more consistent way.

Keep in mind that many books have been written on the topic of thyroid, including our own book, *Thyroid Power*. Our purpose is not to repeat or summarize this more comprehensive information, but instead to provide a sampling of approaches and ideas to help you confront your thyroid challenge in a creative and personal way.

Even though we recommend that you work with a practitioner, we encourage you to make this rebalancing effort a very creative and self-driven process, an honest reflection of *your* own beliefs, visions, and inner guidance.

For some, this will include starting with nutraceuticals. For others, it may mean immediately incorporating specific exercises or yoga postures. Some folks may prefer to start with medication, others with an herbal approach. We encourage you to choose from our suggestions those items you feel are most appropriate for *your* particular situation.

THE AUTOIMMUNE PHENOMENON

There are other ways in which the thyroid is instructive regarding hormone-producing organs in general. An autoimmune thyroid disorder, known as Hashimoto's disease—named for the doctor who first described it—is a common cause of thyroid failure. In fact, scientists now know that the autoimmune phenomenon accounts for most high or low thyroid function. Non-autoimmune high and low thyroid do sometimes occur, but in fairly insignificant amounts compared to the autoimmune variety.

There are many other kinds of thyroid problems. A goiter is thyroid swelling, which can occur from iodine deficiency, or too much cassava (tapioca), which is one of a number of food items known as goitrogens. These are foods that when eaten in considerable amounts (more than the average person with a well-rounded diet might consume) cause swelling of the thyroid gland.

People can have nodules or cysts on their thyroid glands. There can be infection, or trauma, that will affect thyroid function that also is not autoimmune. But in developed countries, these causes taken together still constitute a small number of overall thyroid cases, compared with the overwhelming amount of autoimmune disorders.

It is now becoming apparent that the autoimmune phenomenon is the source of other glandular involvement, not just the thyroid.

The appearance of thyroid autoimmunity should alert both doctor and patient to the distinct possibility of autoimmune glandular involvement elsewhere.

It is quite common to have multiglandular illness, called polyendocrinopathy, a long, hard-to-pronounce word that means there are more than one or two endocrine glands involved with the autoimmune phenomenon at the same time, causing multiple problems for the body and a large variety of symptoms, making it harder to diagnose.

Mild low or high thyroid is often a hidden factor in a person's overall health, and can make any other condition worse. Arthritis or trauma could each be *much* more problematic if the thyroid is off balance and has not been diagnosed. Early identification of thyroid imbalance requires attention to subtle symptoms, suspicions due to family history, as well as looking at lab tests.

A person can be low thyroid despite normal tests because the tests currently used are not sensitive enough to uncover all the people who have this condition.

The best way to improve a thyroid condition is to create your own personalized mix of medicines, combined with carefully selected alternative therapies. Often, taking well-chosen herbal or vitamin supplements as recommended in this chapter can improve your thyroid function if you are not taking medicines, and can improve the effectiveness of the medicines if you are already taking them. And last, since this condition is largely autoimmune, attention eventually must be paid to this phenomenon.

WHY FURTHER BALANCE THE THYROID?

The thyroid gland is the gas pedal for every other organ and every other biological function. Normalizing a thyroid that is too high or too low results in improvement in thyroid-related symptoms. Sometimes there is a total remission of a long-standing problem with this simple maneuver. Helping someone who is thyroid-imbalanced is like offering them a whole new life. The results are frequently dramatic. This helps us to understand why good diagnosis and treatment are so crucial.

Any other illness is worse if your thyroid is off balance.

Body energy and recuperative force will be lower if your thyroid hormone is low. Being too high in thyroid is also unhealthy. It can lead to high blood pressure and heart arrhythmias. It can cause accelerated aging. Most important, it can totally throw off the balance of your other energy and regulatory hormones. Therefore, neither high nor low thyroid hormone levels are desirable. You are looking for good thyroid hormone balance, and this is what will be most restorative.

STRONGER INTERVENTION WITH SPECIFIC NUTRITIONAL THERAPIES

If you are a **physical** endo-type and now want to improve thyroid function beyond the initial vitamins and antioxidants recommended in chapter 5, you may start with some of the stronger items below. Many health food and vitamin stores carry these products, and as mentioned previously, they can easily be ordered via telephone or Web site. Please see page 257 of Appendices.

Taking supplemental nutrients can often improve the function of your glands. While this is our goal, it is best to be aware of symptoms of excess hormone that might arise as your glands improve. For those taking prescription hormonal preparations, we recommend that you have regular medical evaluations (every six months or more often if you begin to experience signs of excess activity—see questionnaires in chapter 3 for symptoms of high thyroid, adrenal, sex-gland output.)

As the glands improve with nutritional supplementation, there may come a time that you need to decrease the amount of your prescription medicine. This is a positive step, because it means your glands are being more properly fed and are working better. This is another reason we suggest you familiarize yourself with the signs of hyperthyroid, hyperadrenal, and excess estrogen or testosterone as outlined by questionnaires in chapter 3).

Finding that exact right amount of nutritional supplements, medicine, and healthy activity for your body is a continuous balancing act. Generally nutritional supplements do not result in excessive hyperfunction of the gland, but instead result in mild symptoms that can be used as feedback to enable you to properly adjust your program.

We strongly advise that you make your changes slowly, starting with one new item, allowing several weeks or up to a month to evaluate its effectiveness prior to adding another change.

Initially, it may not be so critical to limit additions to one item at a time, if you have determined that your body is deficient in a variety of nutrients. However, as you begin to improve, you may want to monitor your progress in a more comfortable and gradual manner. By adding one item at a time, it will be easy to identify and eliminate any undesirable change.

Amino Acids

Specifically, we urge you to concentrate on **taurine.** Beyond what is in the recommended free-form mix, the individual amino acid taurine should be taken as a 500 mg capsule on its own. Include this with your morning vitamins. The extra amount of this one item helps regulate your thyroid amino acid metabolism, which is important for any rebalancing effort.

If you are high thyroid, the amino acid to add in addition to the mixed aminos is **tryptophan,** which was available over the counter until 1989, then was available through prescription only, but has recently returned to over-the-counter status. An additional 500 mg of this item, best taken at bedtime, will help soothe the extra agitation that high-thyroid people often experience. Alternatively, you may simply replace this recommendation with 100 mg of its precursor, 5-hydroxy-tryptophan (5-HTP) sold at most reputable health food stores.

(Tyrosine, another amino acid, is the backbone of thyroid hormone. Contrary to popular belief, it is hardly ever in such short supply that its level would limit the production of thyroid hormone. Therefore, thyroid sufferers do not specifically need to supplement tyrosine just because of their thyroid status.)

Enzymes

In addition to these amino acids—another very helpful early intervention is to take high-quality **digestive enzyme** products. Ordinarily, with a properly functioning thyroid, you would have the metabolic energy necessary to synthesize the protein enzymes that facilitate cell maintenance and growth. If your thyroid is low, your enzyme complement is liable to be low, as well.

You may simply take two capsules of standard, high-quality, mixed digestive enzymes along with each meal, and one pill along with each snack. As your thyroid gland becomes more restored, this maneuver becomes less necessary. Many people rely on digestive enzymes over long periods of time, but we are more cautious, and believe you should take these only initially. Our program is devised to increase the function of specific glands that can improve overall organ function. Enzymes can provide a temporary boost to digestion. We feel that, except for older people, eventually your well-tuned body will be able to properly digest and assimilate nutrients without taking additional digestive enzymes.

Once again, this topic is currently debated among natural practitioners, since some are convinced that due to depletion of our soil, and chemicals that interfere with normal body function, we are unable to make the proper amount of digestive enzyme without additional support. One practitioner in our community uses specific enzyme therapy as a backbone for her program. Ellen Cuttler, MD and licensed chiropractor, worked with Karilee and our daughter over several months in her Mill Valley, California, office, helping to balance the specific enzymes for digesting various types of food intake. She is presently traveling across the United States, teaching practitioners to use her protocols and software for improved results.

Karilee was also treated at the Metabolic Nutrition Center in San Rafael, California. Harold Kristal, DDS, originally a dentist, studied with the nutrition pioneer Adele Davis in 1952, as well as various other reknowned nutritionists, and devised a metabolic typing system that enables people to understand how their bodies metabolize foods, and which foods work best for their specific digestive type. By conducting a series of simple in-office tests, they ascertain one's metabolic type, which is the fundamental way a body produces and processes nutrients. His book, coauthored by James M. Haig, NC (Nutritional Consultant), is called *The Nutrition Solution: A Guide to Your Metabolic Type* (North Atlantic Books, Berkeley, CA). Enzymes were part of his program as well.

In addition to enzymes being responsible for breaking down food in the digestive tract, they are also imminently useful all over the body for maintenance and repair of crucial tissues.

There is another group of enzymes, such as the brand Wobenzyme, that is extremely helpful for generalized inflammation, particularly that resulting from long-term low thyroid. Manufactured in Germany, this product is a *systemic* enzyme formula, where the enzymes are specially coated to pass through the stomach and enter the bloodstream. There they break down harmful proteins that irritate tissues and slow recovery. General dosage recommendations are three tablets twice or thrice daily taken forty-five minutes before meals.

Helpful Herbs

One final group of "nutrients" to consider for thyroid difficulties is the **herbal medicines.** Many of today's commonly used medicines have their origins in herbs. They can safely ease individual symptoms of thyroid problems. Depending on your situation, herbal products can be used to augment prescription medicine if you are already taking some, or to reduce the amount or the need for prescription medicine altogether.

- In general an herbal remedy useful for thyroid symptoms is the common ordinary herb **rosemary.** This is a source of *carnosic acid*, which is absolutely essential for thyroid hormone to do its work, helping to read the DNA inside our cell nuclei. There are products containing this important item, such as Metagenics's Thyrosol or Xymogen's MedCaps T3.
- Another very useful herbal medicine is withania somnifera, sometimes called **ashwagandha.** This unusual-sounding herb is from the pharmacopoeia of ayurvedic medicine of India, and is extremely handy for helping those with thyroid problems convert T4 into T3. Most people in this country take T4 (Synthroid) for low-thyroid problems, yet many of them have problems converting T4 into the active form of the hormone called T3. Ashwagandha is very helpful with this conversion.

    A convenient form of ashwagandha is the Metagenics product Exhilarin. (Two tablets twice daily provides 300 mg of this important root extract.) Xymogen makes a similar excellent product (Med Caps T3, take two daily). Some people who might consider taking the T3 thyroid hormone thyronine (brand name Cytomel) along with their regular T4 thyroid medicine, thyroxine (Synthroid or Levoxyl) could perhaps try this herbal approach first. If the herbal approach works nicely for you, you may not need the additional prescription medicine.

- As Phoebe discovered, one of the most helpful of all herbal interventions for thyroid balancing is the pharmaceutical grade commercial mix of almost two dozen specially grown herbal items from Europe. This product is so effective that in some countries it is a prescription medicine but is available over the counter in North America under the brand name **Padma Basic**. This unusual combination has the distinct ability to normalize autoimmunity, especially the thyroid type. Take two tablets twice daily. (See the EcoNugenics listing in the Appendix section "Locating Your Recommended Vitamins" on page 257.)

- An exceptionally good and more advanced version of immune system rebalancing, particularly for those whose saliva or bloodspot test showed positive for thyroid antibodies, is the **medicinal mushroom** category. These are some of the strongest herbal medicines ever discovered. (For instance, a fungal product that you may have heard of is called penicillin.) These items can be further enhanced with a special growing process, utilizing food nutrients and herbals as a substrate in which they are grown. The product to consider is the Ten Mushroom Formula made by EcoNugenics (see page 257). Take two capsules twice daily for immune normalization.

Iodine

One additional natural item that warrants discussion is iodine. This substance is essential in the production of thyroid hormone, yet even slightly too much, or too little, can cause unexpected problems.

In much of the world, **too little iodine** is a major issue for the population. It causes infertility, miscarriages, birth defects, goiters, and mental retardation, affecting more than one billion people on the planet. In the industrialized countries, the problem was identified and largely handled by putting small amounts of extra iodine in salt and bread dough. Thus, for a long time, **iodine adequacy** was the norm in developed countries. The problem of large numbers of iodine deficiency goiters and retardation seemed to have been eliminated.

Now, however, in certain parts of industrialized countries, we are seeing more iodine deficiency once again. The problem of **iodine**

excess, however, may possibly be an even larger issue for some people. Iodine excess in genetically thyroid sensitive people causes increased autoimmune difficulty. This autoimmune problem is separate from the high-or-low iodine problem, but these issues overlap and influence each other.

In many parts of our country, most people are getting the proper amount of iodine. Others, however, may have iodine excess, and still others have iodine insufficiency. Faced with this problem, the general recommendation has been to avoid anything except the very standard amounts of iodine that are in foods and vitamins. People taking thyroid medication especially may want to avoid extra iodine intake, because thyroid pills already have plenty of iodine in the thyroid hormone they contain.

Our best recommendation is as follows: If you live on or near the coast, and you eat seafood or sea vegetables regularly, and you have a family history of thyroid or other autoimmunity, then you might want to avoid extra iodine. Taking extra iodine might worsen your condition.

If, however, you live in the mountains or the interior of the country, and you're not a seafood or sea vegetable eater, then you may want to use iodized salt or take multivitamins with iodine. This is especially true for the iodine-deficient goiter belt area around the Great Lakes. The amount people need is actually small. A standard multivitamin has about 100 to 150 mcg, which is likely to be plenty for daily intake, according to most scientists. A few researchers are beginning to suggest a large increase in iodine consumption, but the majority of scientific opinion is against this new advice.

Homeopathic Remedies

Another item to consider is **homeopathy.** Once again, we have a whole system of healing devoted to balance, which is what thyroid sufferers desperately need. Thyroid, being the major regulatory gland, is involved in balance of so many body systems that the rebalancing potential of a good constitutional homeopathic remedy cannot be overstated.

Just as with acupuncture, which we'll talk further about in chapter 9, to be good for thyroid, high-potency constitutional homeopathy needs

to be practiced by very skilled, well-trained, and experienced practitioners. The requirements are often very subtle, individualized, and sensitive
to small variations. If you are treated in this way, which we heartily recommend, do your best to find someone who is advanced in his or her
experience.

There is, however, another level of homeopathy that you can incor-
porate into your program on your own.

This is homeopathic first aid. You may purchase low-potency single-
remedy homeopathic medicine from your health food store, as easily as
you buy vitamins and herbs. Very useful for most *low-thyroid sufferers* is
the first-aid remedy Thyroidinum in the 6x or 6c potency. Take three
pellets under the tongue three times daily for one week. For *high-thyroid
people*, your initial homeopathic remedy is Coffea 6x or 6c, taken similarly.
Take three pellets under the tongue, three times daily between meals for
one week, and then stop completely. A homeopathic maneuver of this
sort is like using jumper cables on a car with a low battery. It simply helps
to get things rolling in the short term, and is not to be continued for
months at a time.

CONSULT WITH YOUR DOCTOR TO OBTAIN ADDITIONAL TESTING IF NECESSARY

Suppose you are a definite **physical** endo-type, and you are still suffering with thyroid imbalance despite using many of the natural interventions already mentioned. You might want to consider taking actual
thyroid hormone by prescription. When you need it, there is nothing
like it!

It is, however, a prescription medicine, so you will need to be diagnosed sufficiently for a prescribing doctor to be able to offer it to you.
You know well by now that diagnosing low thyroid as currently practiced
by many doctors is too simple and too imprecise. If you feel you are low
thyroid but have a "normal" reading (TSH between 0.3 and 5.0) on your
TSH test, there are many things you can do that make good sense. First,
make sure you ask for the exact numbers. Then, consider this:

The normal range for TSH testing has recently been changed from
0.5 to 5.0 down to 0.3 to 3.0 by the top medical doctors in the country.

The American Association of Clinical Endocrinology (AACE of Jacksonville, Florida) has developed these new guidelines that many labs have not yet incorporated into their range of normals. *Your doctor and lab may be using old numbers.*

If you have a TSH higher than this (3.8 or 4.1 or 4.7, for example), please realize that your result is now considered by the best specialists as indicative of low thyroid, especially if you have family history of thyroid or autoimmune problems.

What this means is that millions of people who have been told they don't have a thyroid problem might indeed be low thyroid after all. The normal range has been cut in half, and this constitutes major new thinking in thyroid care.

**Realize you could still have a thyroid
abnormality, even with normal tests!**

However, just because one of the thyroid tests has been reevaluated in terms of its range of normal, that doesn't mean that blood testing in general for thyroid is now totally accurate. Even with the new TSH guidelines, and even with some of the more sophisticated standard tests, like Free T3, Free T4, and thyroid antibodies, you might remain in the normal range according to the reviewing doctor.

Yet, you could actually be either borderline high or borderline low in your thyroid balance. This means that in order to obtain thyroid medicine, you may need to advocate for yourself, requesting a clinical trial of prescription thyroid hormone (if you are too low), or a tiny amount of prescription antithyroid medicine (if you are too high).

CONSIDER ADDING YOUR OWN PERSONAL DOSE, BRAND, OR MIX OF PRESCRIPTION THYROID MEDICINES

Suppose you are indeed diagnosed with a low- or high-thyroid situation that needs more than nutritional medicine or complementary therapies. At this point, you will probably receive from your practitioner the following standard advice:

- If you are low, you should start on thyroxine (Synthroid), a synthetic T4 thyroid medicine, and stay on it for the rest of your life. The dose you take will be determined solely on the basis of your blood test results.
- If you are too high, you should do a radioactive iodine treatment to ablate (destroy) the gland. Then you will have to start on thyroxine (Synthroid) and stay on it for the rest of your life. The dose you take will be determined solely on the basis of blood test results.

You need to know that this standard advice is *not* the only sensible way to proceed. There are a variety of other options for both high and low thyroid. We can mention only a few of them here, so we urge you to find an open-minded practitioner who will allow your specific desires and your individual responses to be part of the treatment equation.

Other Types of Thyroid Medicines

For instance, if you're working with an alternative practitioner, you are likely to be started on something other than thyroxine. Many doctors inclined to natural remedies tend to prefer the natural thyroid forms, called desiccated thyroid. This is like the previously mentioned over-the-counter thyroid glandular, but with all the active ingredients left in. Its usefulness for some people exceeds that of thyroxine.

Whether you are started on the natural desiccated thyroid or on the synthetic hormone, it should be *your* choice, a decision made in consultation with your practitioner. We are a doctor–nurse team, in practice for more than thirty years, and we can tell you from our experience that some people do better on one, and some people do better on the other. Neither preparation is optimal for everyone.

There is no way of telling beforehand which type is better for you. Most regular MDs will insist the synthetic form is better because, in our opinion, the pharmaceutical industry has exceptionally good marketing and pays for much of the research that doctors think is unbiased. The "natural medicine" MDs have more confidence in the natural form. It is our firm suggestion that you try first one and then the other, to see which is better *for you*. A proper trial is at least five to six weeks.

There are many differences between natural desiccated thyroid gland prescription medicine and synthetic thyroxine (T4) or thyronine (T3) prescription medicine. The bottom line is that each works best in some people, but not others, and to date, there's no telling why that is. Conventional medical doctors often say that the old-fashioned desiccated thyroid is not standardized in terms of having a consistent dosage of medicine per pill. However, it is the synthetic products that have been more often recalled by the FDA watchdogs for inconsistency of dose.

In general, it seems to be a matter of chance which person does better on which category of thyroid medicine. There is one group of people, however, that often does better on the natural desiccated type. Those who have had surgery to remove all or part of their thyroid gland, or who have had radioactive iodine treatment for hyperthyroidism seem to do much better with some or all of natural prescription thyroid medication.

Whether you start with one of the synthetic forms (Synthroid, Levoxyl, Levothroid, or Unithroid if available) or one of the various natural types (Armour, Westroid, Nature-Throid, Biothroid, Proloid), we suggest that the best beginning for thyroid replacement therapy is to *start low and go slow*. In other words, initiate your therapy with a very small level of medicine; then taper to a higher level depending on how your body deals with it. This is called upward titration, and it's definitely the best way to get started on prescription thyroid.

Starting Your Medicine

A good beginning dose of *synthetic* thyroxine (Synthroid and other brand names listed above) is 25 mcg, the weakest strength made. Your eventual dose of thyroxine, after a few months of upward titration, is generally 88 to 137 mcg per day, best taken all at once in the morning.

A good beginning dose of desiccated (*natural*) thyroid is 15 mg (milligrams, not micrograms as for thyroxine) also called ¼ grain. (A grain is 60 milligrams.) Your eventual dose of desiccated thyroid after a few months of titration is generally 60 to 120 milligrams (also known as 1 to 2 grains). This daily dose is best taken half in the morning, and half later in the day. Many people, however, do just as well taking all their medicine once a day in the morning.

Those who have had their thyroid removed by radiation or surgery often need a higher dose than mentioned above, and they commonly do better—in the long run—with the natural desiccated type, rather than synthetic thyroid. No matter what type you are taking, your optimum dose is always a moving target, rather than being fixed for life. Thus, most thyroid sufferers should check in with their practitioner every six months and be evaluated by physical exam and lab tests at least annually.

Monitoring Your Medicine

If you are wondering whether blood tests are any better at monitoring the progress of your situation than they were at diagnosing it, you are indeed wise. It is a good idea to be skeptical of standard blood tests in diagnosing or in treating the condition. Standard blood tests are unfortunately even less helpful in ascertaining your ideal dose than they are in diagnosing the condition. At our clinic, therefore, we use blood *and* saliva tests, combined with body temperature, ankle reflexes, and especially symptom improvement as ways of monitoring your progress toward determining your best dose of prescription medicine.

Most conventional doctors don't follow upward titration according to symptoms, but instead just follow dictates of the standard TSH blood test. They believe that once your blood levels of TSH return to the outdated broad range of normal (most still use the old range of 0.5 to 5.0), then you are at the "right" dose of medicine, and there you generally stay. This leaves many people still feeling hypothyroid at the end of their doctor's upward titration. If you find yourself in this situation, ask your practitioner to try you out on enough medicine to have the TSH be at the *lower* end of the normal range—then see how you feel.

Some people feel fully well only when they take enough prescription medicine to have their TSH test show slightly below the lower end of normal. (A low TSH result means plenty of medicine; a higher TSH signals the need for more medicine.) This is a standard maneuver in thyroid care at university hospitals, but many regular doctors are unfamiliar with it. We frequently observe the odd situation where the doctor is feeling uncomfortable giving a dose of medicine that finally helps the *patient* to feel comfortable! The doctor's discomfort is entirely due to what we call the tyranny of the TSH test and its supposed accuracy. Your home tests, your basal temperature, and your symptoms considered along with your family history, might be useful items to challenge that excessive faith in the veracity of the regular TSH determination.

Mixing Meds

In addition to either the synthetic or the natural type of prescription medicine, neither of which alone may be great for you, what about combining medicines? A significant percentage of people do not do well with synthetic thyroxine alone. They need something added to thyroxine for full benefit. (The same is occasionally true for natural desiccated prescription thyroid.)

For the synthetic T4 thyroxine prescriptions that are not performing well enough, we often see good results by adding 2.5 to 5.0 mcg of synthetic T3 (thyronine) each day. This is sold as the prescription medicine Cytomel. Medical studies about this maneuver, sometimes poorly designed, are contradictory, but large numbers of physicians who use this combination routinely swear by its benefits over thyroxine alone. Moreover, a great many patients who have been tried on this combined therapy are extremely vocal about its clear increased benefit over thyroxine by itself.

Thus, sometimes mixing medicines works very well. Often, a small amount of synthetic added to the desiccated thyroid (or vice versa) evokes a *big* improvement. If your regular one-medicine protocol is not working sufficiently well, then by all means you and your practitioner should entertain a mix of medicines. These days, blood-pressure treatment, arthritis treatment, cholesterol treatment, and especially psychiatric drug treatment all utilize a mix of prescription medicines for optimal results in most cases. As thyroid treatment is evolving, it is becoming a whole new medical world, and you can be part of it.

For those readers who are pregnant, or are contemplating pregnancy soon, the general rule is to stay on whatever amount of thyroid medicine you were taking when you became pregnant. When women are *seriously* low in thyroid hormone, babies can be born with mental retardation, so we urge those contemplating or in early pregnancy to be well-tested. Herbal medicines and special vitamin supplements are best discontinued during pregnancy, unless you are working with an extremely knowledgeable and careful practitioner.

If you have been trying to become pregnant without success, please realize that undetected low thyroid is a very common reason for infertility. In our practice, we have had numerous examples of women sometimes unsuccessful even after several rounds of fertility treatments, who have gotten pregnant and carried to term once they balanced their thyroid. (One even joked on national television that Dr. Shames "got her pregnant!")

Some women are told to be wary of taking thyroid medicine because it can leach the calcium from bones. This assumption is now outdated. The research on people taking extremely high doses of thyroid hormone is mixed, but it is now known that thyroid pills in appropriate doses are good for your bones. Moreover, it has recently become apparent that the fairly common situation of undetected and untreated low thyroid is a *cause* of bone calcium depletion. We recommend being not too high and not too low with thyroid medication, in order to protect your bones. (For more detailed discussion citing relevant research, please see our book *Thyroid Power*.)

THE BENEFITS OF THYROID BALANCE

One major benefit from thyroid balance is that you become more resistant to standard infections and illnesses. When thyroid is balanced, your resistance is better, and the digestion of nutrients that you need to fight bacteria and viruses is improved.

Let's take a closer look at this benefit of improved digestion for a moment. The organs for digestion and assimilation are sometimes running slowly and not very well when the thyroid is off balance. We depend on our gastrointestinal tract, not only for the assimilation of food, vitamins, and minerals that we take into our body, but also for the proper absorption of herbal medicines and other natural remedies.

You absolutely need your intestinal system to be functioning well to do some of the healing that we are outlining in this program. If your thyroid is off balance, your gastrointestinal tract will be off balance. Getting your thyroid function back to normal will help ensure that the various remedies you ingest will actually be doing the most good for you.

Thyroid balance also helps restore and maintain a balanced intestinal flora. Sometimes the thyroid can be helped by taking a high quality acidophilus product. This is basically a replenishment of some of your friendly bacteria in order to be sure you have the right kinds of organisms to digest your food adequately. Many societies around the world intuitively achieve this goal by ingesting significant amounts of fermented milk products, such as yogurt. Health food stores usually have "live culture" yogurt products in the refrigerated section. High-quality acidophilus capsules are generally kept refrigerated, as well. These are best taken early in the morning, prior to breakfast. Generally one to three capsules per day will suffice.

Perhaps the greatest benefit of all is the normalization of your body weight. Once your thyroid is balanced, you may finally stop that seemingly endless tendency to keep gaining. Now your food plan and your exercise program can start working as intended, so that you can obtain the results other people have received all along. It may not matter so much what diet or body movement you choose. Now that the thyroid is more balanced, it all begins to work better.

There are other reasons why someone might do better with a balanced thyroid. One is that you age less rapidly. You grow older much more gracefully. You look your best and have that glow of health. It can be the difference between being dragged through life, kicking and screaming, versus being carried through it feeling your best.

HOW THYROID BALANCE HELPS ADRENAL AND SEX-HORMONE BALANCE

The adrenal hormones and thyroid hormones are hooked together like a seesaw—often when one is up, the other is down and vice versa. If your thyroid is low, your adrenal levels might be high as a compensation for the low thyroid. Improving your thyroid level will allow your adrenals to relax a bit, thereby stressing you out less.

Another example of a specific interaction would be with the reproductive hormones. If your thyroid has been low for some time, chances are you are not making enough sex hormone–binding globulin. This is the protein that carries sex hormones around in the bloodstream. They are not intended to be floating free; all but a small percentage are carried around on special proteins built to ferry them from one part of the body to another.

If you don't have enough of the binding proteins, more of your sex hormones might be floating free in the bloodstream. This can cause the hormone to diffuse more easily into the tissues. Although that may sound like a good idea, too much of any hormone can be harmful. For instance, too much estrogen diffusing into breast tissue can stimulate that tissue into cancerous changes. Being more balanced in your thyroid can make for less of this problem by having proper amounts of sex hormone–binding globulin. So good luck in having fewer problems and more success, both of which are frequent results of proper thyroid balance.

CONCEPT SUMMARY

1. The thyroid gland commonly experiences early failure, due to the autoimmune phenomenon.

2. The appearance of low or high thyroid should alert both doctor and patient to the distinct possibility of autoimmune glandular involvement elsewhere.

3. Another reason for balancing the thyroid is that no matter what your other illnesses are, those conditions are much worse if your thyroid is low.

4. The American Association of Clinical Endocrinology's (AACE) new range for TSH testing is 0.3 to 3.0. If you have a TSH 3.0 or higher, especially with family history of autoimmunity or low thyroid, you should be considered and treated as a low-thyroid patient.

5. Synthetic forms of thyroid medicine include Synthroid, Levoxyl, Levothroid, Unithroid, and Cytomel. Natural desiccated types include Armour, Westroid, Nature-Throid, Biothroid, Proloid. Neither the natural nor the synthetic thyroid replacement is right for every person. Some people do better on natural, some on synthetic, some on a combination of the two.

6. Improving digestion helps with increased thyroid balance and with increased resistance to infections. You can start this process by

adding live-culture acidophilus to your pre-breakfast regimen, and high-quality enzymes before meals.

7. Even though you may work with one or more practitioners (which we heartily recommend), we encourage you to make this rebalancing effort a very creative and self-driven process, an honest reflection of *your* own beliefs, visions, and inner guidance.

ACTION SUMMARY

❑ Add to the prior chapter's suggestions two 500 mg capsules daily of the amino acid *taurine*.

❑ Add a well-chosen mixed *digestive enzyme product*, two taken with each meal and one with snacks. Also consider taking *Wobenzym* as directed for inflammatory process, three tablets twice daily taken forty-five minutes before meals (see "Locating Your Recommended Vitamins," page 257).

❑ The herb *rosemary*, a source of carnosic acid, can be very important for thyroid binding in the cell nucleus. Take 100 mg of a standardized leaf extract daily. The most handy source of this item is the product *Thyrosol* or *MedCaps* T3 (see above Appendix section, page 257).

❑ Take two tablets once or twice daily of the herbal mix *Padma Basic*. (see above section, page 257).

❑ *Ashwagandha* is an excellent adaptogenic herb, or tonifier, that helps in the conversion of T4 to the active form of T3. Take 100 mg of a standardized root extract daily.

❑ *Iodine* can be a double-edged sword for **physical** endo-types, occasionally useful and occasionally precipitating a worse thyroid problem. If you live on or near the coast and you eat seafood or sea vegetables regularly, and you have a family history of thyroid or other autoimmunity, avoid any extra iodine. If, on the other hand, you live in the mountains or the interior of the country and are not a seafood or sea vegetable eater, choose the iodized version of salt, and take multivitamins that include iodine.

❑ *Homeopathic first aid* can be very helpful for initiating thyroid rebalance. For low thyroid, try *Thyroidinum* 6x or 6c, three pellets under the tongue three times daily for one week; and for high thyroid, consider *Coffea*, in 6x or 6c potency, three pellets under the tongue three times daily for one week.

❑ Take two tablets daily of an over-the-counter *thyroid glandular*, regardless of whether or not you are on prescription thyroid medicine.

❑ If you start with synthetic thyroid without good results, next ask for a trial of *natural prescription thyroid*. If you first take natural prescription thyroid without good results, then ask for a trial of the *synthetic*.

❑ When synthetic thyroid prescriptions (Synthroid, Levoxyl, or Levothroid) are not performing adequately, try adding 2.5 to 5.0 mcg of synthetic T3 (*Cytomel*) daily for a few weeks' trial. If it helps, stay on it longer term.

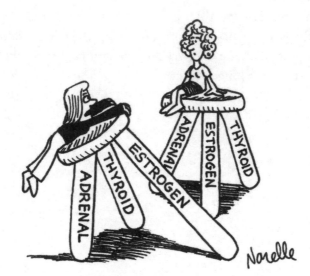

**The doctor says if I don't feel better
soon he'll increase my estrogen.**

CHAPTER 7

IMPROVE FUZZY THINKING: RESTORE SLEEPY SEX GLANDS
Progesterone, Testosterone, and Alternative Therapies

> And to deal plainly, I fear I am not in my perfect mind.
> —William Shakespeare

You'll recall that Meredith is the well-organized single mom whose memory had recently become a problem. After going off birth control pills, adding some simple nutritional items, and eating fewer hidden hormones by purchasing organic meat and poultry, she began to notice improvement. Her program had so far resulted in slightly improved mental clarity. She then called for a phone coaching session to help her figure out how to proceed.

She was still having trouble with water retention and breast tenderness. All of this was in spite of her recent increased ability to follow conversations and remember grocery lists much more easily than she had previously. Nevertheless, she still had severe estrogen dominance, and happened to be a person who was especially sensitive mentally to her estrogen levels.

After we reviewed her situation and tests, Meredith was presented with a choice of whether to use natural remedies only or to combine those with prescription interventions. She clearly needed some progesterone to counter the estrogen excess. This item is available in prescription or over-the-counter forms; therefore, we asked what she preferred.

After the negative experience with prescription birth control pills, she readily chose to start with a nonprescription form of progesterone. We recommended an over-the-counter natural progesterone cream, sold under the brand names Progest or FemGest. She purchased this item and begun using it right away, much to the trepidation of her teenagers, who were concerned that mom would once again get worse. In spite of their fears, after only a couple of weeks of twice daily application of ¼ teaspoon of the topical cream, Meredith began to see even further improvement.

She was able to think through problems much more easily now. Missing a meeting at school or a luncheon with friends had become a thing of the past. Breast swelling and water retention both eased.

She was much less spacey, foggy, and no longer felt disconnected. Yet she was not all the way better. The water retention and breast discomfort, although better, had not resolved completely. It appeared to us that she was having a processing difficulty with estrogen metabolites, where the discomfort is more often a result of the breakdown products on their way to being removed from the system. We suggested another simple intervention.

The results were dramatic. After only one week on a health-food-store item called I-3-C, which readjusts metabolites to a more benign ratio, she felt totally like her old self. It worked miraculously, and she was happily relieved.

WHY FURTHER BALANCE SEX GLANDS?

Most people would be quite surprised to learn the extent to which the reproductive hormones are involved with proper brain function. Brain processes related to memory and intellectual capacity are stimulated by the sex steroid hormones, which include estrogen, progesterone, testosterone. It has long been known that abnormalities in the levels of these hormones are associated with mood alterations such as dementia, anxiety, and depression. Less well known is that the difficulties that people experience with fuzzy thinking and memory challenges are frequently related to their sex-hormone balance.

Many entire books are written on this subject. Our goal in this chapter is not to repeat, duplicate, or summarize those efforts. (Some of these books are listed in our Further Reading section for your added exploration of this vast topic.) Our purpose is simply to present a representative sample of the variety of useful tools you might utilize for immediate rebalancing, if you are the **mental** endo-type. Your job is to choose from this list of tools what you feel is most appropriate for *your* particular situation at any given time.

Also, considering the complexity of these sex-gland hormones, we have focused on estrogen and progesterone for women and testosterone for men for purposes of simplicity. We do want you to be aware that both sexes have all three of these types of hormone, and in certain instances men benefit from exploring their estrogen or progesterone levels, and women may need fine-tuning related to their testosterone. Generally, however, that is not the case, so we are simplifying the steps in this manner.

The reproductive hormones are responsible for one's sharpness or edge. They control mental spark in general and one's mating behavior in particular.

Perhaps there is a good reason for this connection. To mate well requires a presence of mind, a certain sharpness, a focus of desire. This might be why the reproductive hormones are so connected with intellectual capacity.

Whatever the reason, it is this intellectual ability that often suffers first when the reproductive hormones are slightly off balance. Nor is it just estrogen we are talking about. Abnormal levels of testosterone are associated with unfocused thinking and depression in men. Low levels of progesterone are associated with anxiety and difficulty with focusing in women.

Of course there are a host of other reasons for wanting to rebalance your sex hormones. These include having a healthy sex desire, normal reproductive tissues, and strong muscles and bones. These regulatory hormones affect a great many activities throughout the body. Your intellectual function might be a barometer of this balance, and it is better for the whole body when you are less fuzzy in the head.

So let's bring this spark alive. Let's create more of this edge, sharpness, and focus in your life. Balancing your sex hormones is like turning on your car's ignition. The spark ignites your engine. As we improve the brain's ability to hum along, that will help in healing all aspects of the body tissues, as well.

STRONGER INTERVENTION WITH SPECIFIC NUTRITIONAL THERAPIES

Nutritional and herbal supplements that you can buy without prescription can influence the level of your individual sex hormones. You need to do this very carefully, and you really ought to have a qualified practitioner to guide you. Just as with thyroid balancing, you are free to try nutritional interventions on your own, but may do better with a knowledgeable and supportive practitioner. This might be your family MD, naturopathic physician, chiropractor, acupuncturist, nurse practitioner, or licensed nutritionist. Please see our Appendix section called "Finding Appropriate Practitioners" for additional help in finding a friendly practitioner locally, or consider a telephone coaching session with Dr. Shames. (Go to www.FeelingFFF.com, or call 866-468-4979.)

Sometimes, it is very difficult to find just the right practitioner to work with you in this way. Although some health providers are willing, many of them do not have the skill, expertise, or time to become as knowledgeable in this area as is necessary. Thus, it is occasionally justified for you to make the initial forays into rebalancing sex hormones on your own. This can be done safely and sensibly, as we describe below.

First, one preliminary rule. You need to avoid so-called brain stimulants like ephedra or guarana. These products seem to help give mental clarity initially, but then they drop you like a hot potato and you crash. The end result, in the long run, is that you are actually worse off than before. Also, you may become partially dependent on the substances. This will not be at all helpful for your focus and concentration and memory. You should even begin to view caffeine more as a stimulant of last resort, with proper hormone balance gradually providing the main strength for getting through your day.

Severe calorie-restrictive dieting is also a problem. When you start starving yourself, the first place that often gets starved is the brain, and then you have less spark, less focus, and less concentration than you had before.

If you are the **mental** endo-type, one of the specific nutritional interventions that might be helpful for you is *amino acid therapy*. The sex gland type of person has foggy thinking and less mental sharpness, often because abnormal levels of sex hormones interfere with the neurotransmitters in the brain. These are the chemicals that encourage the nerve conduction flow across the empty space of the synapse.

With good neurotransmitters, you can think more clearly and more effectively. If your sex hormones have altered the neurotransmitter balance, it is often in the direction toward less catecholamines. These are adenaline, noradrenaline, and dopamine which help with energy and alertness.

You can restore the flow of catecholamines with 500 mg twice a day of the amino acid *tyrosine*. This is the building block for these neurotransmitters, and the inclusion of it in your program could be quite safe and beneficial for more clear thinking.

People who are the **mental** endo-type might have increased difficulty at various certain specific times of their lives. The woman who is younger might have PMS-type symptoms, a woman who is a bit older might have perimenopausal problems, and an older woman might have postmenopausal issues. For each of these specific situations there are individual over-the-counter remedies that we will recommend. Infertility, recurrent miscarriage, pregnancy, and postpartum difficulties are special situations requiring a variety of additional nutritional and herbal interventions. There are many books written specifically outlining herbs that can or can't be taken during pregnancy.

If You Are the **Mental** Endo-Type with HIGH Estrogen (for Women)

Overall, be aware that too much estrogen causes water retention; breast enlargement; irritability; anxiety; and, in certain sensitive women, fuzzy thinking

---

Women with the highest levels of estrogen in their bloodstream sometimes have the lowest levels of cognitive function.

Causes of High Estrogen

What could be causing such high levels of estrogen? It is known that a diet high in soy products could give you a fair boost because of the amount of phytoestrogens that it would contain. Other sources of phytoestrogens might increase the uncomfortable estrogen effect. People may not realize that birth control pills cause a significant estrogen increase in many women, even though this medication is usually a combination of synthetic estrogen and synthetic progesterone.

The environmental factor cannot be overstated. There are a great many xenoestrogens (unintended estrogenic chemical pollutants) in the environment. These could have two distinctly undesirable effects. One would be that overall you are more estrogen dominant, because these compounds (insecticides, herbicides, fungicides, and so forth) are having an estrogenic effect on your body. If this alone isn't bad enough, long exposure to some of these may cause an actual decrease in the follicle function in the ovaries. Because xenoestrogens are largely environmental in origin, you need to become aware of what you can do to avoid and counteract them.

Recall that the ovarian follicle is where an egg matures and is then released. After releasing the egg, the follicle now starts to secrete progesterone, for the continued safety and care of the egg as it moves into the uterus for implantation. Without a properly functioning follicle, the postrelease secretion of progesterone is severely diminished. A woman whose ovarian follicles are burnt out by "environmental estrogen" becomes progesterone deficient, causing further estrogen dominance.

Helpful Solutions for High Estrogen

All of this is generally tackled first with *natural progesterone*, which can balance out the effects of estrogen dominance and can be purchased over the counter. Progesterone is a calming agent that provides a sense of greater relaxation; too little progesterone can cause feelings of anxiety.

This is your primary maneuver and is possibly all that you will need. We recommend progesterone cream in the standard over-the-counter potencies. Ten to 20 mg rubbed into the upper body once or twice a day does wonders. It may even help an overly estrogen dominant woman to conceive that baby she has been wanting, if she takes the progesterone in the twelve days before menses.

In addition, you can eliminate estrogen by preventing the body's natural recycling process. A great deal of your metabolized estrogen is taken out of the bloodstream and goes into the gastrointestinal tract as part of normal metabolic activity. This might ordinarily be removed from the body, but instead, an enzyme reactivates some of the spent estrogen for reabsorption. The recycling process often accounts for 30 percent or more of the total estrogen in your body. *Calcium deglucarate*

(CDG) is an over-the-counter nutritional product. Taking 400 mg twice a day with meals can block some of the reabsorption enzyme activity. Regardless of the cause of the estrogen excess, reducing the amount recycled is often helpful.

Also a good high-quality fiber supplement (we use OptiCleanse by Xymogen and MetaFiber by Metagenics—blend, shake or stir one level scoop into your favorite liquid daily—see Recommended Vitamins section) might be additionally helpful for binding up the extra estrogen in the intestinal track. Daily routine use of a sensible fiber supplement would be a fine idea for most people on a typical city-dweller diet. This will not impair, but rather help, your body's natural ability to eliminate. You can also focus your food selection to include higher-fiber foods so that eventually you may not need to take fiber supplementally, though it is not a problem to continually supplement with fiber products that do not contain laxatives.

The next item that you can utilize to your advantage would be *to improve your liver function* with even more of the specific antioxidant, *alpha-lipoic acid*, 100 mg twice a day. Add to this 100 mg of *methionine* and 500 mg of *n-acetyl cysteine*. Next, add 250 mg each of *inisotol* and *choline*, special B-complex vitamins. This will help your liver's ability to deactivate estrogen.

Limiting alcohol, a known liver irritant, to a maximum of two drinks daily will help your liver to stay healthy. (A drink is equivalent to 1.5 ounces of hard liquor, one can of beer, or a glass of wine.)

Another item also sold over the counter *for estrogen excess* is *indole-3-carbinol*, abbreviated I-3-C. Four hundred milligrams a day is very effective in transforming some of your estrogen into its friendly, easily tolerated metabolites, instead of the more toxic ones.

We've mentioned it before, but it seems to bear repeating: If you suspect you have multiple gland involvement, start rebalancing the most troublesome gland first, as determined by self-evaluations and testing. Many times, tackling the worst symptoms first, alleviates some of the minor symptoms, as well, eliminating the need for more specific rebalancing of the other two legs of the stool. Do your best to ascertain which problems need to be addressed first, and proceed cautiously for several months on just those new protocols, so that you do not overwhelm your system. If later you feel you need additional help, you can try rebalancing the secondary gland.

Keep in mind that sometimes the situation of estrogen dominance is not so much an oversupply of estrogen, but instead that there is too little progesterone to counter the normal amount of estrogen that exists. This is, as mentioned above, generally well handled by increasing the amount of natural progesterone to counter estrogen dominance. This condition may show up on your self-evaluations as too much estrogen. Actually it may be simply too much estrogen "effect," which would mean not having enough progesterone. Either way, progesterone cream is a good bet for most women.

Another helpful product is dong quai, an herbal medicine that is a great balancer, and a tonifying herb. A daily dose of 150 to 300 mg is often quite helpful. It has the property of cooling things down if you are too high in estrogen. Ironically, it also can heighten a situation that has been too low in estrogen. This means that dong quai is in the category of herbal medicines that are adaptogenic, able to work in either direction depending upon the person's needs. This leads us into the next section, which explains how to boost estrogen if you are too low. Dong quai, generally used in combination with other herbs, falls into both these categories.

The adaptogen herbs are usually quite safe. Like any of the items we mention, however, they have the potential in some people for mild temporary adverse effects. The type of symptoms from these rare side effects varies greatly from person to person. Our best advice is for you to immediately discontinue anything that has the bad manners to disagree with you in any way, and to be especially cautious regarding pregnancy.

If You Are the **Mental** Endo-Type with LOW Estrogen (for Women)

The symptoms of too little estrogen can be moodiness, sleep difficulty, decreased memory, mental fogginess, and—as if all this wasn't enough— difficulties with sexual function.

Not having enough estrogen makes you sleep less, which adds to the foggy brain problem.

There are a variety of maneuvers that are relatively benign and easily available over the counter for improving your estrogen level if it is too low. These natural maneuvers may be preferable to taking estrogen itself.

Why not just take estrogen if your levels of it are low? After all, this was until recently the most common prescription in the world. "It looks like you are low in estrogen. Here's your prescription for Premarin." Probably many women reading this book have heard that advice.

Karilee was astounded when, after a satisfactory checkup at a new gynecologist's office, the nurse practitioner handed her a bunch of small sample boxes on her way out. "What's this?" she asked. "Estrogen," was the response. "But, we never discussed this," Karilee said in confusion. "Don't you care about your heart and bones?" the nurse practitioner asked, as if that were all there was to discuss.

Within a year after this experience, the Women's Health Initiative Study was halted due to the results showing that not only was estrogen *not* protecting women's hearts and bones as much as was initially suggested, but in addition, it was increasing the chances of cancer and other serious health problems. Subsequent studies have validated that concern. Thus, we urge you to look at natural options first.

- You can simply go to the health food store and get *black cohosh*, and/or *chasteberry* (Latin name *Vitex agnes*), common and widely used herbal medicines. (Be especially sure to use either of these two only as long as you're certain you're not pregnant or trying to become pregnant.) They have a definite estrogenic potential that often helps a person who is dealing with the foggy thinking and fuzzy brain of a low-estrogen **mental** endo-type.

There are other herbal medicines that can be used for safe and mild estrogen boosting:

- In addition to dong quai mentioned earlier, the Chinese medicine pharmocopeia has popular formulas called Two Immortals (or its variant, Three Immortals) that are estrogen-enhancing herbal mixtures.

- A North American herbal mix that would have a similar salutary effect on a low estrogen system might include motherwort, licorice, alfalfa, red clover, and pomegranate. These are all weak estrogens that could be helpful to you.

- Of course, you could also try increasing your intake of soy products, as long as you do not have a thyroid problem. (Recall that too much soy can slow down thyroid activity. See below.) The isoflavones in soy are mildly estrogenic. Since they are plant-derived, they are known as phytoestrogens. One substance that might cause a problem is the soy isoflavone genestin. This happens to also be a mild goitrogen, meaning it can reduce thyroid function or even promote unusual growth of the thyroid gland, called a goiter. (If you want to see how much soy might be appropriate for your specific situation, review the more detailed soy discussion in the "things to avoid" section of chapter 9.)

Sometimes your low sex-hormone situation, especially low estrogen, might simply be the *lack of production*. This can occur when there is not enough adrenal strength, since the adrenals make a large amount of the sex hormones. For women, that is especially true after the ovary decreases estrogen output at perimenopause. You can increase the amount of the raw material that the adrenals would have on hand to work with to promote the likelihood of your body making more estrogen if you are low.

One way to accomplish that goal would be to take pregnenolone, which is a precursor to adrenal and sex hormones. This increases your adrenals' supply of raw material, which can improve adrenal function, leading to better support of estrogen levels. Good adrenal precursors, such as pregnenolone, are available at high-quality health food stores. As always, we recommend starting one item at a time, slowly, and monitoring progress prior to adding other items. You might start with *25 mg of pregnenolone, increasing gradually* over weeks if your body accepts this adjustment well, moving to *50 or 100 mg a day.*

If your trial of pregnenolone is not sufficiently beneficial, another precursor to estrogen is DHEA. This is an abbreviation for dehydro epiandrosterone, an intermediate substance that is further along the metabolic pathway producing sex hormones. If you are low in estrogen or testosterone you may want to consider taking DHEA, starting with 5 or 10 mg. If this step proves successful, you can slowly titrate up to 25 mg a day. Remember pregnenolone and DHEA are effective hormone building blocks, even though they are available over the counter.

They should be used sparingly and cautiously, until their benefit and comfort to you have been established. Remember to *start with* one at a time, not both, and if they make you feel worse for any reason, just stop taking them. If you feel better after your initial trial, it's fine to continue taking them together, even long-term if needed.

(Note: Women under thirty-five probably do not need DHEA unless their tests show a marked deficiency. *Pregnant or nursing women should avoid DHEA altogether.*)

Also available are a number of vitamin, mineral, and herbal combinations in the form of *prepackaged medical foods*. These high-level nutritional products, which are more like "nutraceuticals" than vitamins and minerals, are sometimes available only through working with a practitioner. Several highly regarded companies make various formulas that can be mixed with juice or into a shake for morning consumption. One of those is called Estro-Balance (by Metagenics) or MedCaps PMS (Xymogen), which includes many of the items already mentioned—to have things be a little more in tune with each other. Our Recommended Vitamins section lists several highly regarded companies that manufacture medical foods.

Perhaps the best way to achieve balance with your hormones is with the generalized balancing intervention of one of these medical foods, rather than trying to figure out which hormone is high or low and then intervening precisely to affect only that hormone. The overall approach has a lot to commend it. We encourage you to call or visit the Web sites listed at the end of this book for high-level nutritional products, and to experiment until you find items that really resonate with your body. Remember to be patient and to pay attention; start one product at a time, give it at least a couple of weeks before adding others, and regularly evaluate how you're feeling and what you are noticing.

For this purpose we once again recommend that you keep a journal or notebook of your trials, symptoms, and successes or failures. It will be very helpful for keeping track of what works for you and what doses are effective.

Sleep Concerns

If you are having the difficulty of high or low estrogen, with the resultant effect of a reduced ability to sleep, that could be due to decreased levels of serotonin. Sleeplessness often occurs at PMS time or at perimenopause and menopause times.

Helpful for these sleep disorders is *the amino acid 5-hydroxytryptophan, abbreviated 5-HTP*. It is available at health food stores and is a *precursor to serotonin*. Taking *100 to 300 mg* of the amino acid often helps to improve sleep. Taken *at bedtime*, it can give you a wonderful night of restful restorative sleep instead of time spent tossing and turning. This simple over-the-counter product might be more effective and less addictive than prescription sleeping medicines. Also, it is less expensive than actual tryptophan.

Another beneficial item is angelica. Angelica is an herb root that is very helpful in estrogen balancing, especially for women in a young age group, perhaps thirteen to thirty-five years. For slightly older women, thirty-six and over, and especially menopausal women, a useful item is the herb macca, which has been a source of healing in South America for centuries. Grown high in the Andes, macca is very helpful for a variety of menopausal symptoms, including sleep problems. It is also recommended for women who have breast cysts or tenderness.

These are merely a few items that might be helpful in balancing your estrogen, which in turn will help to regulate and improve your brain function.

If You Are the **Mental** Endo-Type with HIGH Testosterone (for Men)

Your body can get ahead of itself by producing too much testosterone. Although not a commonly diagnosed condition, excess testosterone is by no means a rare phenomenon. Some studies of prison inmates find consistently high levels of this one hormone in the most violent offenders. If you couple violence with illogical, fuzzy thinking, then you may have the formula for quite a bit of the criminal behavior resulting in incarceration. Too much testosterone can cause accelerated loss of hair, acne, oily skin, bossiness, aggressive behavior. Thus, being at a better balance with your testosterone is highly important.

Testosterone seems to help with stamina and muscles, controlling body fat, maintaining strong bones, promoting physical and mental strength, helping you to feel more stable and have an appropriate sex drive.

To help with a reduction if your testosterone is too high, try to *find out why the levels are high* in the first place. (If you are taking the supplement DHEA, maybe that is not what you need. This pro-hormone often becomes estrogen and testosterone.)

To further reduce testosterone, consider adding *calcium degluterate or indol-3-carbinol,* mentioned earlier on page 131. Whatever reduces estrogen might possibly also reduce testosterone, since estrogen and testosterone exist in relation to each other. So feel free to try these in a careful way (200 mg CDG, 200 mg I-3-C) to see if they help you to reduce the symptoms that result from too much testosterone.

An herbal remedy useful in this regard is *saw palmetto.* You may have heard of its use for treatment of men with prostate problems. One of the ways it helps alleviate their symptoms is by reducing excess testosterone. Regardless of whether or not prostate is an issue for you, the product may be helpful for improving your memory, if testosterone is too high.

Another useful remedy in high-testosterone situations is the *mineral copper* which works in conjunction with zinc and requires a balanced ratio. Try 1 mg daily above what is in your multivitamin/multimineral mentioned in chapter 5.

The most beneficial *amino acid* for you at this point might be GABA (gamma-aminobutyric acid). This product relaxes the extra irritability and anger associated with too much testosterone. Try 500 to 1,000 mg at bedtime.

For the excess testosterone situation use rose aromatherapy. Granted that a person with high testosterone is least likely to stop and smell the flowers, it is worth a try. The aroma can be a body scent or infused into a room. The actual rose flowers are also a fine idea, as is rose-scented bath oil. It can be diffused into your car while you are driving, either via rubbing into cloth or using a car aromatherapy diffuser, purchased at health food or aromatherapy stores.

You might be able to find rose aroma in natural shaving or aftershave products, or even in deodorants, but only at a good health food store. We're not talking about neurotoxic synthetic scents, but rather aromatherapy-grade essential oils from a reputable manufacturer. You might at first write this off as a "feminine" suggestion, but realize that this maneuver may help your out-of-balance body to rebalance. (It is important that you do not use aromatherapy liquids under the tongue, unless you are working directly with a highly trained aromatherapist.) Liquid aromas are very strong medicine, most often meant to be smelled via spray infusion into the room. Certain ones can be applied to the skin, while others may burn skin. It is best to consult an aromatherapy book or expert prior to using scent remedies.

Speaking of flowers, the actual *Bach Flower Remedy* that can counter many of the effects of high testosterone is vervain. You can purchase flower remedies at many health outlets or specialty shops. The proper procedure is to take five or six drops of the liquid remedy under the tongue several times a day, or mix in drinking water that you sip on throughout the day.

An even stronger intervention is the *homeopathic remedy* bryonia. This remedy has the nickname of "the bear" when used for acute upper respiratory conditions, since the indication for choosing it is when the person is vocally and vociferously demanding to be left alone and undisturbed. With testosterone excess, the person frequently acts that way, and the remedy is similar to ameliorate these symptoms.

Homeopathic remedies are recommended taken under the tongue, between meals, and allowed to dissolve. We recommend a 6x or 6c potency, three pellets under the tongue two or three times daily for a week and then discontinue. It is best used initially just to get things moving.

If You Are the **Mental** Endo-Type, with LOW Testosterone (for Men)

What are the signs of testosterone deficiency? Look for a decrease in body hair, a reduction from what you are accustomed to. You might have a decreased sex drive or be more indecisive than in the past. In addition to not being able to make up your mind easily, there is a sense of less security, less coordination, or less strength. You can feel generally less "solid." Longstanding testosterone deficiency might be difficult to notice, as these same symptoms may have been present for so long.

In men, testosterone is helpful for improving memory if one is low in it. Testosterone developmentally increases the size and the number of neurons. It engenders a more determined, steady state of mind, for greater attention and recall.

There is also a lack of endurance or stamina for those with unbalanced testosterone levels.

If you are low in testosterone, one of the over-the-counter items you can utilize is *DHEA, 5 to 10 mg daily*.

(Note: Generally, people under thirty-five and men fighting prostate cancer should not take any form of DHEA at all. You want to avoid DHEA if you have too much testosterone.)

There are a few other herbs, vitamins, and minerals that might also help:

One would be Korean ginseng. Panax ginseng, as it has also been called, has been found in double-bind studies to *result in better abstract thinking and faster mental reactions in those taking it*. It is a brain booster for central nervous system function if reproductive hormones are off.

The herb Withanea somnifera, mentioned in chapter 6 as ashwagandha, an adaptogen, has also been helpful for hormone-related decrease in memory. It has an influence on cholinergic and GABA receptors in the brain. Thus, in addition to the effects it has on helping the thyroid conversion from T4 to T3, it does seem to have several beneficial effects on the central nervous system. Try 600 mg daily.

Another good balancing herb for **mental** endo-types is *bacopa, in a* *standardized extract of 160 mg one to two times daily*. Bacopa has been used extensively as an ayurvedic medicine to help manage cognitive and learning defects. There are published clinical trials with both animal and human subjects that support the herb's application in improving memory.

The key *mineral* for low testosterone is *zinc*. Twenty-five milligrams, in addition to whatever is in your multivitamin/multimineral combination, would be of substantial benefit.

Pumpkin seeds, also known as pepitas, roasted or seasoned, are a fine addition to any meal or snack, with 1 tablespoon being the amount to include in your daily intake to counteract low testosterone.

Homeopathic testosterone in 6x or 6c potency is a strong intervention, as well. Use three pellets under the tongue three times daily for three weeks, and then stop. This treatment is a one-time effort—if it is not successful, do not repeat.

The *aromatherapy* you are looking for in this situation is *sandlewood*.

The *Bach flower remedy* is *mustard*, helpful for low testosterone symptoms, several drops under the tongue or in your water three times daily.

These are some additional things a person suffering low testosterone could try that are available for easy purchase over the counter. Lifestyle modifications can help, too, as you will see in the next section.

CONSIDER ADDITIONAL SEX-GLAND TESTING IF NEEDED

If you have tried most or all the suggestions above, and are not doing as well as you would like, perhaps it is time to consider taking some *prescription medication*. Prescription medicines can come in a variety of forms.

Estrogen, progesterone, or testosterone are all available as pills, gels, transdermal skin creams, sublingual drops, suppositories, vaginal creams, or lozenges.

The type of application you use depends upon personal preference and your practitioner's knowledge. Here are our suggestions:

First, assess how well your program is doing in terms of hormonal balance with the over-the-counter nutritional items and self-care activities. If you seek even greater balance in these hormones, a practitioner can assist you by providing more expert consultation and assessment, including blood tests and twenty-four-hour urine determinations.

Note: Even if you have derived substantial benefit from efforts on your own with the questionnaires, saliva testing, and over-the-counter remedies, you may still want to have a practitioner evaluate your progress to make sure you're on the right track for the long haul. You can have a practitioner review your saliva tests with you, suggesting additional ones to further evaluate your status. If your practitioner is not fully licensed to prescribe, you may need to work in conjunction with a licensed practitioner who can order tests and prescriptions.

Tests to Consider

What are some of the additional tests your doctor might prescribe, or you may want to ask for? The answer depends largely on the type of practitioner you have. If you have a willing partner for a practitioner, who does not routinely test blood for hormone balance but is interested in helping you, then you may want to mention and discuss some of the tests below. Have your practitioner order the estradiol or testosterone saliva test as part of your overall home testing for thyroid, adrenal, and sex hormones.

If on the other hand you are dealing with a seasoned practitioner who has been using saliva or blood hormone testing for years, let him or her guide you to the next level of necessary testing.

Regarding our specific recommendations for more thorough evaluation, we suggest you discuss the following with your practitioner:

Standard blood tests for reproductive hormones. For women, we recommend a blood-estradiol level on day three if menstruating, anytime if not. For men, we recommend a free and total testosterone test. More complete is for men and women to have both estrogen and testosterone blood tests.

To define your estrogen levels more precisely, if needed, the Great Smokies (see below) blood lab can also *fractionate the estrogens*, so that each of these items can be replaced individually. This test determination includes levels for estradiol (the most potent estrogen), estrone (potent precursor to estradiol), and estriol (a more benign metabolite of estradiol).

In addition to estrogen and testosterone levels for both men and

women, there is also a *progesterone level for both men and women* to consider, if you require further refinement in testing. Menstruating women
should have this drawn on day twenty of cycle. Menopausal women using progesterone and men can have it drawn any time. Menopausal
women not taking progesterone are always low.

If taking action based on the above results still hasn't given you the
improvement you're looking for, a further refined measurement would
be the *sex-hormone binding globulin (SHBG)*. This test, seldom ordered, is
occasionally very useful.

The activity of a hormone that is measured in the blood but active in
the tissues is dependent on the levels of the binding protein that carries
it. Just as we discussed in other chapters, thyroid function suffers when
there is too much thyroxine-binding protein; similarly, sex hormone
function will suffer if the levels of sex hormone–binding globulin are too
high or too low. Such a situation can occur regardless of how normal the
blood test level of the hormone might be.

For menstruating women who are wondering if menopause is a
cause of their symptom picture, it can also be helpful to know the level
of *follicle stimulating hormone (FSH)* and *lutinizing hormone (LH)*. These
pituitary hormones control activity of ovarian secretion of estrogen and
progesterone. Increased levels of LH or FSH indicate menopause. Another pituitary hormone is *prolactin*, sometimes ordered to further check
pituitary and sex-hormone functioning.

In addition to the commonly run blood tests, urine determinations
for sex hormones are employed by some practitioners as a further diagnostic refinement. Though this result is debatable, many different estrogen metabolites (breakdown products) and other sex-related hormones
can possibly be more accurately measured from their urinary output.

One of the more sophisticated determinations that you and your
practitioner might find useful is the *estrogen metabolism profile* to see how
your body is breaking down the estrogen it uses. Some breakdown products are more damaging than others. Recall the earlier discussion of the
over-the-counter product indole-3-carbinol (I-3-C). This substance can
help to divert estrogen metabolism toward more benign breakdown
products. Estrogen metabolite testing is a way to determine for sure if
such a product would be helpful or necessary for your optimal balance, if

the lab is chosen carefully. We only use GSDL for this kind of work. (See Great Smokies Diagnostic Laboratories in lab test section of the Appendices.)

After more thorough testing (if needed and agreed upon by your practitioner), you will likely be moving toward a more fine-tuned balance. Many women find out that they have satisfactory estrogen levels but low progesterone. You can be advised further on how to use natural progesterone under guidance of your practitioners. There are a variety of good methods for bio-identical progesterone, in the form of creams, gels, pills, or lozenges.

Realize you could still be low or high in sex-gland hormones *even* with normal tests!

Keep in mind that even the best reproductive hormone blood or urine tests may not show mild imbalance. Remember no matter how much testing you do, you may still have a medical problem and show on tests as quite normal. Since lab tests reign supreme in today's medical system, many practitioners will treat hormonal situations only if tests are outside the normal range.

Remember, you can still be abnormal on sex-hormone balance even with normal tests, particularly if they are blood tests. What you do with that information is up to you.

If your symptoms are severe enough to warrant it, you and your practitioner may want to consider prescription hormone intervention even though tests don't show abnormality. This is called a therapeutic trial. If you are better, that's great. If not, hopefully it was worth a try. Such a trial should start with small amounts of the hormonal medicine in question. The rule once again to follow is "start low, and go slow." If you don't notice improvement at the lower dose, then gradually move up to a higher dose. If a problem develops, go back to the lower dose or discontinue entirely.

Next, you should reevaluate the situation often to properly monitor your progress. The way to evaluate your progress is to see how your mental clarity is doing. Do you feel sharper? More focused? How is your overall mood? These differences, even if small, may indicate that you are on the right track. If improvement is great, they can indicate that you are now on the correct amount of estrogen or testosterone.

If instead you feel you are getting foggier, along with experiencing vaginal dryness or hot flashes, you may be too low in estrogen. If you are bloating, feeling foggier, retaining water, and have tender breasts, then you may be on *too much estrogen*.

How well are you sleeping? If you are having restless nights, and trouble falling asleep, then *maybe you do not have enough estrogen*. Are you getting more uptight and irritated? This may indicate too much estrogen, or too much testosterone.

As you can see, some of the symptoms listed are similar to symptoms for the other glands; for this reason, it is ideal to work with a seasoned practitioner to determine how to treat your hormone imbalance.

CONSIDER ADDING YOUR PERSONAL DOSE, BRAND, OR MIX OF PRESCRIPTION SEX HORMONES

Progesterone

Keep in mind that progesterone cream, while an over-the-counter product, is still a very strong intervention. Using transdermal hormone creams can result in high levels of progesterone. In such instances, saliva tests may show a ridiculously large measurement. A very high progesterone level means that you are using too much of the cream. The amount you need for feeling less fuzzy is actually quite small.

The standard good-quality over-the-counter cream has about 900 mg of natural bioidentical progesterone for every 2 ounces of cream. A measured dose of approximately 20 mg once or twice daily has been the commonly recommended dosage. One quarter to one half of this dose is usually quite sufficient to reestablish mental clarity in most people who are thinking fuzzily because of estrogen dominance. The better-quality preparations are packaged with a metered way to dispense accurate dosage.

You and your practitioner may want to have progesterone cream "compounded" just for you, in the right strength and the most pleasing form. This customizing can easily be done by consulting with one of the many excellent "compounding pharmacists" all over the country who are—like holistic doctors and nurses—breaking out of the old molds and creatively practicing the art and science of pharmacology. They realize that many people with these subtle gland imbalances are very sensitive, and sometimes react to additives and fillers in the standard pharmaceutical products. Simply using individually compounded natural cream bases instead of "one size fits all" medicines can make a world of difference in your comfort and ability to utilize the hormone. Most medications can easily be compounded into natural bases for greater comfort. (See the "For More Information" section for compounding organizations.)

Where you apply the cream is important. The upper body has thinner skin, so the hormone cream is more uniformly and consistently absorbed there. Natural bioidentical micronized progesterone also comes in standard-sized pills or they can be made up in any size by a compounding pharmacy. Many women use pills that are from 50 mg all the way up to 200 mg daily.

Estrogen

When it comes to estrogen, you can be given pills or creams, as well. Always insist on *bioidentical hormones*, which are closest to what your body makes naturally. The situation with estrogen can be quite personalized, since there are many kinds of estrogen.

The most common kind of bioidentical estrogen used in pills is estradiol, or E2. It is a potent estrogen, but can also cause troublesome side effects.

Another kind of estrogen is estriol, or E3. This estrogen is more benign and milder than E2, but you may need more of it to achieve the same therapeutic effect.

You can obtain both these estrogens combined as *Bi-Est* (bi-estrogen creams or pills). The preparation is usually 20 percent E2 (estradiol) and 80 percent E3 (estriol). With the very potent estradiol present in only small amounts, you have greater safety with similar efficacy. Bi-Est is an evolution from the previous Tri-Est formulas, which used 10 percent estrone (E1), 10 percent estradiol (E2) and 80 percent estriol (E3). Tri-Est is now less popular than its variants since estrone seems to be associated with increased side effects, and therefore it has fallen out of favor with some practitioners. Using more than one kind of estrogen at a time is a more sophisticated approach than simply taking 100 percent estradiol, as in an Estrace pill.

Combined E2 and E3 estrogen may also be *wiser than taking Premarin*, which is a non bio-identical mixture of many different estrogens from pregnant mare urine. It has lately been discovered that two of the horse estrogens are actually chemicals that women's bodies have never tried to metabolize, and may act like a metabolic monkey wrench for some. Thus, the horse chemicals may not be as sensible an approach as Bi-Est.

Similar concerns might lead a thoughtful woman to avoid the progestins (the term for synthetic progesterone), Provera and Norlutate. These are *synthetic look-alikes* to real progesterone. As altered forms, they can be patented and sold at a higher price than the genuine bioidentical progesterone, which cannot be patented.

Testosterone

Men, please see the action summary at the end of this chapter for specific recommendations for high and low testosterone.

HOW BALANCING SEX HORMONES HELPS THYROID AND ADRENAL

We know that estrogen is anti-thyroid, due to the fact that the more estrogen increases, the more there is thyroxine-binding globulin (TBG) in your bloodstream. This substance ties up thyroxine so it can't go into tissues where you need it. Your blood tests may look good, but you may feel bad anyway. Keep in mind that we live in an overestrogenized society, which is one reason why we currently have so many thyroid problems.

As far as adrenal function is concerned, reproductive hormones are intimately involved. First of all, the adrenal gland is the source of much if not most of our sex chemicals as we age. If your adrenal is producing lots of cortisol (because it is continually stressed), you may not have enough adrenal power left over to make your sex hormones.

If you are the *mental* endo-type, you need to balance your sex hormones carefully even if you are not having difficulty with typical sex-gland symptoms or cycles.

If you are having some other "typical" sex-gland symptoms (such as low libido, hot flashes, or bad PMS), then be sure to find your way to balance. Even though other hormones and nutrients are involved with memory, the sex hormones are a good place to start. Addressing sex hormone dominance or deficiency will help your thinking and will improve your chances for better weight and mood, as well.

CONCEPT SUMMARY

1. The reproductive hormones control one's mental spark in general and one's mating behavior in particular. Too much estrogen causes water retention; breast enlargement; anxiety; and, in a few very sensitive women, fuzzy thinking.

2. If high in estrogen, reduce soy products, birth control pills, and xenoestrogens from your environment as best you can. You can also benefit from adding natural progesterone creams to counterbalance excess estrogen. If you are pregnant or trying to become so, do not attempt hormone balancing except on the advice of your personal practitioner.

3. You can interrupt estrogen recycling to slow down its increase. You can also benefit from cleansing the liver with specific nutrients; this liver cleansing topic is explained in many excellent books on detoxification (see the "Further Reading" section of the Appendices).

4. You may not be making enough estrogen if you have decreased adrenal power. *Too little estrogen* can cause moodiness, sleep difficulty, decreased memory, mental fogginess, and sexual function issues. You can increase your estrogen by taking precursors to adrenal and sex hormones.

5. Testosterone helps with stamina and muscles, controlling body fat, maintaining strong bones, promoting physical and mental

strength, and general well-being with appropriate sex drive. Too much testosterone can cause accelerated loss of hair, acne, oily skin, bossiness, and aggressive behavior.

6. You could be low or high thyroid, adrenal, or sex hormones *even with normal tests*. We recommend follow-up testing if needed, possibly a therapeutic trial of hormone to see if it helps improve your most uncomfortable symptoms.

7. Both men and women can benefit from using bioidentical hormone preparations to help with the symptoms of sex-gland imbalance, which is preferred to any synthetic or equine estrogen mix. Maintaining balance among all three energy hormones allows for your greatest health.

ACTION SUMMARY

HIGH Estrogen

❑ Avoid brain stimulants and severe calorie restrictive diets.

❑ 500 mg of the amino acid tyrosine helps restore neutrotransmitter function.

❑ 5 to 20 mg natural progesterone cream (ProGest, FemGest) can be rubbed into the upper body once or twice a day to counter excess estrogen. To minimize estrogen recycling, add 400 mg CDG (calcium deglucarate) twice daily with meals, and also begin taking a daily fiber supplement.

❑ Improve liver function with more of the costly but highly beneficial antioxidant *alpha-lipoic acid* (100 mg twice a day). Add to this 100 mg of *methionine* and 500 milligrams of *n-acetyl cycteine*. Next, add 250 mg each of *inositol* and *choline*, the special B-complex vitamins. These can sometimes be found combined in one tablet. Limit your alcohol intake.

❑ *Add indole-3-carbinol* (I-3-C), 400 mg a day, to change estrogen into the more friendly, easily tolerated metabolites instead of more toxic ones.

❑ Add some dong quai, a tonifier and adaptogenic herb.

LOW Estrogen

❑ Always use herbal remedies with the advice of your practitioner. To boost estrogen, you can use herbal remedies such as black cohosh, chasteberry, Two (or Three) Immortals, motherwort, licorice, alfalfa, red clover, and pomegranate. Increase soy as long as you don't also have low thyroid.

❑ If lowered adrenal function is causing lower estrogen, consider introducing pregnenolone, precursor to adrenal and sex hormones, start at 25 mg per day, increasing over weeks to 50 or 100 mg.

❑ If pregnenolone doesn't quite do it, try adding DHEA, a precursor to adrenal hormone that is further along the metabolic pathway, starting at 5 to 10 mg per day, gradually increasing to 25 mg. Only start *one* new product at a time! Also keep in mind that DHEA is generally more effective at increasing testosterone in men than increasing estrogen in women.

❑ For disrupted sleep, try the *amino acid 5-hydroxytryptophan, abbreviated 5-HTP, a precursor to serotonin,* at bedtime. Taking *100 to 300 mg* of this amino acid often helps improve sleep. If 5-HTP is not fully helpful, replace it with actual tryptophan, which has recently returned to the market. Use 500 to 1,500 mg.

❑ For breast cysts or tenderness, try the herbs *macca, angelica, or vitex.*

HIGH Testosterone

❑ To reduce excess testosterone, eliminate DHEA if you are taking it, and add *calcium degluterate (CDG)* or *indol-3-carbinol (I-3-C).* (While not proven to be as effective for high testosterone as for high estrogen, they are worth a try.)

❑ In addition, add the *herb saw palmetto* for decreased testosterone and improved memory, the *mineral copper* (1 mg above what is in your multivitamin/multimineral), and the *amino acid GABA.*

❑ For gentle balancing support, use *rose aroma* for high testosterone, and add the *Bach Flower remedy vervain,* plus *the homeopathic remedy bryonia.*

LOW Testosterone

❑ Helpful remedies include DHEA, Korean/panax ginseng, Withania somnifera for CNS symptoms, and bacopa for cognitive defects.

❑ Add 25 mg zinc, above what is in your multivitamin/mineral combo. Also it's good to munch on pumpkin seeds daily for extra zinc.

❑ You can also try the *homeopathic testosterone in 6x or 6c potency*, the *aromatherapy sandlewood*, and *Bach flower remedy* of *mustard*.

❑ If testosterone is low and estrogen is normal or high, ask your doctor about the prescription medicine Arimidex, which inhibits the conversion of androgens into estrogens. Dose is 1 mg once daily.

Adding Bioidentical Hormones

❑ *Progesterone:* A standard good-quality over-the-counter cream has about 900 mg of natural bioidentical progesterone for every 2 ounces of cream. Apply a measured dose of approximately 20 mg once or twice daily. Apply on the upper part of the body for greater absorption. Pills of 50 to 200 mg daily are another option.

❑ *Estrogen:* The most common kind of bioidentical estrogen is estradiol (E2). Estriol (E3) is more benign and milder, so you need more of it. Bi-Est (combined E2 and E3 as compounded pills or cream) is an often helpful and sophisticated approach, especially when E3 is 80 to 90 percent of the total.

❑ *Testosterone:* The bioidentical hormone cream, either brand-name prepackaged or individually compounded, is available like estrogen—only by prescription. For mild testosterone boosting in men, use 1 to 3 g daily of a 1 percent cream.

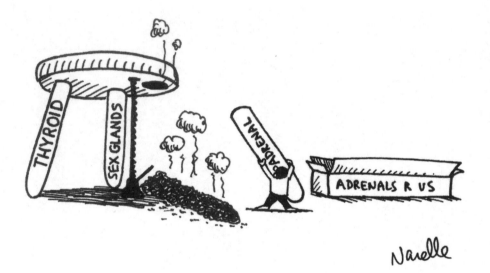

CHAPTER 8

ELIMINATE FRAZZLE: REBUILD BURNT-OUT ADRENALS
Pregnenolone, Glandulars, DHEA, and Cortisol

Six o'clock. The burnt-out ends of smoky days.
—T. S. Eliot

Recall that what helped Emily, our ambitious but frazzled young stock-broker, to start feeling better was a high-potency multivitamin with minerals. She also eliminated coffee and artificial sweeteners, and added a brisk nongoal-directed walk twice daily, along with changing from slow floor exercises to the much more active salsa dancing. This worked better to release built-up agitation than her old exercise regime.

Happily, after following a few of these general suggestions, Emily was beginning to feel slightly improved. So encouraged, she was eager to embark on a more definite and specific rebalancing program.

We then advised her to take fairly high doses of extra vitamin B_5 and B_6 along with her multivitamin, which already contained a mix of B vitamins but not in these specific higher amounts. Because her saliva test results showed the typical second-stage adrenal-insufficiency with high levels of cortisol in the evening, we suggested she also take one pill of SeriPhos at bedtime. [This specially phosphorylated brand of the nutritional amino acid serine is one of the few over-the-counter items that can help reduce excessive cortisol. (See page 251.)] Lower evening cortisol often helps a Stage II person to sleep better. Because her tests, taken at various times throughout the day, showed low levels of cortisol in the early morning, we recommended that she take two

*tablets of Licorice Plus, a high-potency licorice extract (see page 160)
first thing in the morning.*

*The addition of these two supplements evened out her sometimes too
high, sometimes too low variation. Since cortisol is the main stress response hormone for daily life, she was now much more comfortable both
at home and at work. She seemed less on edge, more able to respond appropriately with her coworkers, who then found her easier to deal with.*

*Although she felt better, Emily was still not back to her "normal" self.
At a follow-up appointment, she asked what else could help restore her
previous calm and centered style. At this point, we suggested that it was
time to start deep-tissue bodywork. This would allow her to free up some of
the excess tension in her muscles, tendons, ligaments, and joints. It could
also provide emotional release that occurs when painful tissues are stroked
harder than the typical "relaxing" massage.*

*Emily, now highly motivated, jumped into this suggestion whole-
heartedly and saw beneficial results right away. This was the proper rebalancing medicine for her, and before long she felt much better.*

WHY FURTHER BALANCE ADRENALS?

If you are an **emotional** endo-type, you have a magnificent challenge. The
adrenal is one of the most complex and misunderstood glands in the body.
A surprising amount of benefit will reward your rebalancing efforts.

Once again, there are several excellent books written on this adrenal
topic alone, as listed in our Further Reading section. Our mission in this
chapter is not to repeat or summarize those efforts, but instead to share
a sampling of helpful approaches you might choose to utilize for immediate rebalancing. Rather than a prescription or protocol, consider this
chapter a menu from which you may pick and choose interventions that
feel most appropriate for *your current* situation.

**Even though you may work with one or more
practitioners (which we heartily recommend), we encourage
you to make this and any other hormone rebalancing
effort an honest reflection of *your* own beliefs,
visions, and inner guidance.**

Adrenal Structure and Function

Part of the complexity in rebalancing your adrenals is that the adrenal is really two glands in one. There is an outer cortex that secretes hormones known as corticoids (such as cortisol, sometimes called hydrocortisone), which control a wide variety of body processes that keep maintaining normal function during times of stress. Corticoid activity involves responding to stimuli, in other words, dealing with the outside world. Regulation occurs on an hourly or daily basis. There is also an inner core of the adrenal gland, called the medulla, which secretes hormones called amines, such as adrenaline.

The medulla hormones manage our response to external stress on a second-to-second or minute-to-minute basis. For instance, the fight-or-flight action of adrenaline occurs almost instantaneously. This response is life-saving when threat is imminent.

A problem arises when a threat, or stress from the external world, is no longer imminent, short term, or quickly resolved. Short-term situations were common for our distant ancestors who lived a more simple life. After running away from a bear or chasing after a lizard for food, there could be a relatively long period of rest and recuperation. Now times are different. These days, stress can be ongoing, stretched out over days, weeks, or months.

The adrenal gland controls body fluid balance, blood pressure, blood sugar, and other crucial actions. It provides a tremendous amount of immediate energy to deal with a threat or to escape danger. Increases in blood pressure and heart rate help the body to move quickly. Other cortex hormones, called glucocorticoids, mobilize extra blood sugar and bring up additional immune reserves. This type of activity is essential to proper function for anyone except those sitting on a couch watching television all day. If there is no stress to handle, you may not require much in the way of adrenal function.

The Stress Response

Keep in mind that sometimes stress is self-generated, such as that which occurs when our emotions (fear, insecurity, anxiety) overwhelm our ability to function well. The tension and anxiety people feel from internal stress can be ongoing and long-term. The physiological state resulting from ongoing stress can result in adrenal excess. If it persists long enough, the situation can cause the adrenals to burn out. This condition has other causes than simple long-term stress.

The adrenal gland has a very peculiar way of slowing down when it has been overtaxed and overburdened. It fails in the manner of a large dying star, which gets brighter and brighter before it burns out.

At first, the failure causes an increase in the production of certain adrenal hormones, resulting in a hair-trigger release of chemicals even with a mild stimulus. In addition, there is longer duration of response. This particular way of winding down by first cranking up is not unusual in biological systems. It does, however, make evaluation and treatment a little more tricky.

The three stages of adrenal insufficiency were first elucidated by Hans Selye, MD, a pioneer in the field of stress and stress response. He called these stages the general adaptation syndrome or GAS. Indeed, what happens when the adrenal glands fail is akin to a car running out of gas.

1. The first stage is called *alarm*. This occurs when, for instance, a car backfires and you feel "rattled" for several minutes. Why does this happen? The adrenal gland releases an inordinate amount of hormones in response to the perceived stressful event. Even if you do become excessively rattled for several minutes afterwards, things settle down and you are basically a normal person until the next stressful event.

2. Second stage adrenal insufficiency is called *adaptation*. Here, just the routine activities of daily life are enough to trigger an excess adrenal response. For example, having to stop at a stoplight that you wanted to go through could result in an inordinate amount of anger. It might be worse if someone cuts you off at an intersection. Events that would not generally be considered stressful at all are now evoking a strong reaction. Almost everything now is causing a higher-than-normal secretion of adrenal hormones.

   People going through this stage have an edge to them that

others don't understand or appreciate. This fairly common second stage of adrenal insufficiency is what many practitioners, and patients, call "high adrenal."

Moreover, continually bathing the tissues in high levels of cortisone results in cell damage, and eventually cell destruction. This makes you prone to a variety of illnesses, including increased blood pressure, increased kidney ailments, and greater strain on the heart.

3. The third stage of adrenal insufficiency is *exhaustion*. Here, the adrenal gland is depleted and no longer producing sufficient amounts of hormone for daily life. A person in this stage is not as able to mount a fight-or-flight response. Sometimes they know this, and run their life so as to avoid as much confrontation as is possible. When they do meet up with stress, it throws them into significant physical and mental difficulties, such as illness or depression.

What this can mean to you is simple.

Without diagnosis and treatment, adrenal insufficiency can create havoc in your life. It is difficult to evaluate properly because of the various different stages involved.

Often a person who is in one stage can be confused with being in another. Blood and urine testing are not always accurate for determining whether you have the condition—*or* which stage is actually troubling you.

Part of the extreme difficulty in dealing with the diagnosis or treatment of these various stages of adrenal insufficiency is that the adrenal medulla may not be failing at the same rate as the adrenal cortex. Frequently a person will not have enough cortisol, but will have plenty of adrenaline. The medulla may be overpumping, as if it is in stage II. The cortex may be totally exhausted in stage III. So the result now is too much adrenaline and not enough enough cortisol, making you high and low at the same time, which can be very uncomfortable and difficult to diagnose.

A person who has a high level of adrenal hormones is sometimes properly advised to increase exercise, as this will help burn off some of the excess adrenaline. Although this works perfectly for some people, others who follow this advice might be heading for worse problems. Exercising when you don't have the cortisol and other glucocorticoids (hormones that control carbohydrate metabolism) and mineralocorticoids (hormones that control kidney metabolism) can further deplete the system and throw things even more off balance. Often, a nutritional intervention is a better first choice.

BOOST ADRENAL POWER WITH NUTRITIONAL THERAPIES

Sometimes adrenal insufficiency can be a result of autoimmune impact, or toxic pollution. Stress can combine with toxic load to produce a marked decrease in adrenal function. Often, adrenal imbalance requires the help of a high-level practitioner, though occasionally it can be managed on one's own. If you are an **emotional** endo-type, based upon self-evaluations and home tests, you might initiate some of the simplest adrenal rebalancing steps by yourself and see how it goes. Adrenal is one gland that, when altered, can quickly make you feel really good, or really miserable.

If an **emotional** endo-type moves toward an eating plan that includes high-quality food taken in small frequent meals, that person is doing his adrenal gland a favor. It is best to choose foods that are easy to digest, nutrient-rich, and contain a mix of carbohydrate, protein, and "good" fat each time you eat. In fact, if you eat consistently six small meals a day instead of the regular three, that will be exceedingly helpful for your adrenals. The adrenal-driven person, often low in some needed enzymes, finds it much less stressful to eat lightly and more often, as well as having each meal be a comfortable balance of different nutrients.

Now for a surprising recommendation: Adrenal difficulties are often helped by salt. If you have a salt craving, that might mean that you have an adrenal problem, and this is one case where you can rightfully succumb to the craving.

You might try using sea salt from a health food store. This is generally better than regular non-iodized or specially iodized salt, both of which are available at grocery stores, and which could be a problem if you have a coexisting thyroid situation or are allergic to iodine or both. The sea salt is best because it contains a wide variety of helpful trace minerals. Although there may be some small amount of iodine naturally occurring in sea salt, it is not as potentially harmful as the specifically iodized salt, which is intended for people living inland, in an iodine-deficient area (the Midwest or Great Lakes).

*Extra salt can be good for **emotional** endo-types.* The admonition to avoid salt is generally for the minority of people who have a problem with salt affecting their blood pressure. Many people in the population who have the adrenal-driven endo-type should have more salt intake, not less. If you are a thyroid sufferer taking thyroid medication, the extra salt used would best be noniodized. When adrenals are depleted, the kidney does not receive enough hormonal instruction via the adrenal hormone aldosterone to retain salt that is needed to run the body. This problem can be handled by taking in more salt with the diet. Not long ago, in fact, salt was one of the treatments recommended by medical doctors for adrenal insufficiency. Today they give prescription forms of the hormone or hormonelike substances themselves.

Check your blood pressure. Generally people with adrenal insufficiency have low blood pressure. Often they run 100 over 60 or less. If you are the **emotional** endo-type and if your blood pressure is normal or especially if it is low, try using extra salt for a few weeks and see how you feel. Eat salty foods if you like them, and use the salt shaker at every meal. At the end of this little experiment, notice if you are feeling better, and also regularly check your blood pressure to make sure it is not too high (no higher than 135 over 85).

People vary widely in terms of their major problematic substances. For Emily, as you recall, salt was not important, but caffeine was a big problem. This is a question of individual differences. Many **emotional** endo-types are utilizing—to their detriment—caffeine, alcohol, tobacco, sugar, and chocolate. In the final chapter of this book (chapter 12) we explain more about how and why to avoid these.

Adrenal-driven people often crave these substances because of the low energy and uncomfortable feelings that accompany their metabolic imbalance. If you are in this situation, you will do better to somehow decrease the amount of problematic substances in your life. Your adrenal glands can heal, and give you their best, but you must first give them a fighting chance.

In addition to the major recommendations above, many people simply need more of a few very specific vitamins and minerals:

Adrenal-gland processes involve **pantothenic acid.** This is not really much of an acid. It is actually vitamin B_5. This particular vitamin frequently does an absolutely beautiful job boosting low adrenal activity. It is a commonly used item, but many folks use far too little of it to derive supportive benefits. Most **emotional** endo-types need as much as 250 mg two to three times daily.

The addition of vitamin B_6 to the B_5 gives a synergistic effect that neither one of these vitamins alone is able to provide. An extra 50 mg of B_6 two to three times daily is generally a godsend when it comes to boosting adrenal function.

In addition to the above recommendations for general care and feeding of adrenal metabolism, there is a specific nutrient for the sometimes-difficult Stage II situations. (Recall that this is when your cortisol levels might be too low at one part of the day and too high at others). **Phosphorylated serine** (we use SeriPhos brand, a 1,000 mg capsule to be taken once or twice daily) seems to have the beneficial effect of decreasing cortisol levels when they are too high. (This is not to be confused with phosphatidyl serine, a very similar-sounding nutritional product that has very different uses.)

First check your saliva test to see which time of day your cortisol level was too high. Now try taking 1,000 mg of phosphorylated serine an hour before. Do this each day for a week, and see if you feel better.

When your cortisol levels are too low all day long (such as occurs in the third stage of adrenal insufficiency), the use of the herbal medicine **licorice** can be most beneficial. Licorice is one of the few herbal medicines that acts like a hormone-mimic in the body. It increases cortisol levels in a somewhat similar fashion to the way that Prozac increases serotonin levels, by increasing cortisol activity at its binding sites.

When we describe licorice extract, we are *not* talking about the candy or the tea. Nor are we describing deglycerized licorice, known as DGL, which is helpful for discomforts of the intestinal lining. We are talking here about full-strength licorice extract, unaltered. The active ingredients, glycyrrhizin and glycyrritinic acid, have been studied sufficiently to qualify them as strong interventions with dramatic effects. In fact, licorice is so strong that people with high blood pressure are admonished not even to eat licorice candy.

We recommend that you start with 300 mg daily of the actual standardized licorice root extract containing 12 percent glycyrrhizin (usually the dose of one pill). Each week, you may increase by an additional pill until you are taking three or four pills each day. Be sure to check your blood pressure each week during this tapering up phase.

All in all, the use of licorice for people who are low in cortisol has had amazing benefits at our clinic. It is one of the most effective items we know of for natural adrenal support.

Depending on your success with licorice, other effective items for adrenal balance can easily be added. Most notable among them are the **adaptogenic herbs.** As you may recall, the adaptogens are special herbal medicines that have the ability to readjust biological systems either up or down, depending upon what is needed. If things are a little low, they bring them up; if things are high, they bring them down.

This is known in the herbal field as tonifying. Natural items that tonify are called tonic herbs. A tonifier seems to exert its influence by functioning at the binding site of the hormone itself. In the case of adrenal hormones, the receptor binding sites are throughout the entire body. Rather than increasing the amount of hormone floating through the bloodstream, the usual action of the tonic herbs is to adjust the hormone receptors.

For instance, if you consider the hormones as keys floating in the bloodstream seeking their respective locks, then the tonifiers are agents that tighten or loosen the locking mechanism. The tonifiers help the process achieve greater balance either by speeding up or slowing down the binding process.

Many other herbal and chemical medicines used for hormone-balance work by increasing or decreasing the amount of hormone present in the bloodstream. The adaptogens, as you can see, work in a very different and useful way.

One example of a well-known adaptogenic herb is **ginseng,** which is also a tonifier. It will boost certain functions and lower others. For this reason, ginseng is particularly useful for adrenal situations. Be aware of the various types. Asian ginseng (*Panax ginseng*), available as pills, powders, or liquid, is the one that seems to be most generally helpful for cortisol and adrenaline balance. The amount we recommend for the average person is 400 mg daily of a root extract, standardized to 8 percent ginsenosides.

In addition to ginseng, one of the more well-rounded and multiuse tonifiers is **ashwagandha.** Good for both thyroid and adrenal, its benefits are well documented in the health literature. Either with or without ginseng, ashwagandha at 600 mg per day could be a welcome addition to your adrenal program.

If you have not derived as much benefit as you would like from the above adaptogens, there are quite a few others. Some of the more useful ones for **emotional** endo-types are

- **Cordyceps,** 800 mg daily cordicepic acid standardized 8 percent extract,
- **Rhodiola,** 100 mg daily standardized to 1 percent salidroside, and
- **Bacopa,** 500 mg daily of a leaf extract standardized to 16 percent bacosides

These are very common herbal remedies used worldwide, but they are not well known, or much utilized in this country.

Perhaps more common than taking adaptogens is the use of over-the-counter hormone precursor items that actually increase the body's supply of the needed hormone. This maneuver is called precursor augmentation. A precursor is an earlier step in the assembly phase of the needed hormone.

For instance, the precursor of many adrenal hormones is **DHEA** (dehydroepiandrosterone). This chemical is sold at health and vitamin stores, but is a very potent medicine that should be used cautiously. **Emotional** endo-types often benefit from taking 5 or 10 mg a day. That is a small amount compared with the amounts recommended at times by lesser-trained salespeople.

Occasionally a higher dose of 25 to 50 mg per day is indeed recommended by natural practitioners, but only after a very careful evaluation, and an upward titration. If your estrogen and testosterone levels are low on the saliva test, then adrenal boosting with DHEA might be a very good idea, because it is also involved in earlier stages of the production of sex hormones.

Even more of a precursor is **pregnenolone,** which was mentioned in chapter 7 for women with inadequate estrogen production. It is an even-earlier step in the production of adrenal hormones. It is sold over the counter and used by the body to make DHEA. Unlike DHEA, however, pregnenolone can actually become aldosterone and cortisol. If your cortisol levels are low and the herbal items are not helping enough, you may want to try the addition of 50 to 100 mg of pregnenolone daily. Sometimes this treatment will make a major difference in your adrenal function, allowing you to feel better.

This is, of course, assuming that the adrenal gland has enough productive power and is healthy enough to make use of added precursors. Sometimes, however, the problem is in the capability and enzyme-power available for the assembly phase. In such situations, it may not matter how much of the precursor you have. You may need to actually add something more akin to the hormone itself.

There are a couple of different ways to do this. One method is to take **natural adrenal gland** substance (desiccated gland). This is very similar to taking natural thyroid glandular, as mentioned in chapter 6. The adrenal glandulars are sold over the counter and are made from animal adrenal gland.

A careful start of one pill every other day, followed later by one per day, might be a good way to begin. Some people have an increased reaction to the sometimes unavoidable adrenaline-like compounds that get into the glandular when the inner medulla gets mixed with the outer cortex in the process of making a two-part animal gland into a pill. Many people get a little bit "speedy" from the adrenaline, nullifying the benefits of the cortisone-boosting aspects. If you are tolerating the pill well, but still want to increase the dose, you can slowly work your way up to three to four pills daily.

A higher-quality version of this glandular approach is the Bezwecken product **IsoCort.** This is a very useful and purified adrenal glandular that many doctors and clinics find superbly helpful for their patients, available through Bezwecken in Beaverton, Oregon. Adrenal glandulars vary greatly in strength and consistency; this one brand appears to be more uniform than some others. To obtain it, however, you will likely need to be working with a licensed practitioner.

Another way to support your adrenal power is to use **adrenal glandular liquids,** sold in dropper bottles at health food stores. A stronger version of glandular liquids is sold by compounding pharmacies, available by prescription.

A third way would be to use **homeopathic adrenal.** Usually the 3x or 6x potency is utilized, and three pellets are dissolved under the tongue three times daily for three weeks. Then be sure to stop. We repeat, homeopathics are not ongoing medicines in the same way as are vitamins or herbs, given that they work to stimulate certain aspects of your life force, then allow the body to take over in better balance.

Stronger adrenal balancing is available by prescription. A later section of this chapter shows you how to work with your doctor for additional testing, if necessary, and additional prescription medicine, such as physician-grade cortex extract, or the pharmacy version of hydrocortisone itself.

CONSULT WITH YOUR PRACTITIONER TO OBTAIN ADDITIONAL TESTING IF NECESSARY

If you have not received as much benefit as you would like from the natural and over-the-counter remedies that we have described above and you are a definite **emotional** endo-type, you may want to ask your medical practitioner about further treatment for your imbalance. You can present what you've done so far and then ask for some specific additional tests of your adrenal status. Of course, you can still have mild abnormal adrenal function even if these more rigorous tests look normal. Consider them merely as a way of trying to check more carefully.

Ask for a twenty-four-hour urine sample to measure cortisol and DHEA. You can also get a blood sample for cortisol and DHEA. Insist on a free and total cortisol, with DHEA-S (DHEA sulfate), which are more accurate versions.

The *timing of the blood cortisol test for the adrenal is crucial.* Standardized times are 8 a.m. and 4 in the afternoon. Make sure you have the tests done at both of those times and only at those times. Also try to have the blood draw performed on a typical stressful workday, rather than when on vacation.

If you are a particularly stressed person, another standard test to ask for is a twenty-four-hour urine (or a one-time blood sample) for catecholamines. This will generally include adrenaline, noradrenaline, and dopamine. This test, however, is often read as normal, even for an extremely agitated person, because of an overly wide normal range.

The reason to ask for this test is that sometimes it does show an elevation, and this can be convincing for a practitioner who otherwise would not believe that you have an adrenal problem. However, a "normal" result may not tell the whole story.

The same is true for adrenocorticotropic hormone (ACTH) measurements. The idea here is to see if cortex hormone levels are so low that the pituitary (which secretes ACTH) is asking for more output from the adrenal gland. This situation does occur in the rare instances of Addison's disease. ACTH levels in Addison's are high, suggesting adrenal levels are low. But Addison's disease is merely the most extreme form of a wide spectrum of adrenal insufficiency.

Sometimes a more sensitive test than ACTH is needed. This is called the ACTH stimulation test. It is intended to *measure adrenal reserve,* which is believed by some practitioners to be a more sensitive measure of mild adrenal insufficiency. Well before a frank adrenal insufficiency occurs, there is a period of decreased adrenal reserve.

The method is to stimulate the adrenal cortex with a shot of synthetic ACTH, measuring cortisol levels immediately before the shot, and an hour afterwards. Once again, however, this test has a wide range of normals, and you could still be abnormal even when the test shows you're fine, depending on who interprets it.

Realize that you could still have abnormal function
even with all the blood tests showing normal.

CONSIDER ADDING YOUR OWN BEST DOSE, BRAND, OR MIX OF ADRENAL MEDICINES

Generally people do not need prescription medicine for the kind of adrenal balancing we are discussing in this book.

When it does become necessary to treat for adrenal deficiency with something beyond over-the-counter medicines, the first choice is **cortisol** itself. A more familiar name for this compound is hydrocortisone, available at drugstore as an over-the-counter 1 percent cream.

The cream is usually used for the itching of poison oak and eczema. This same exact medicine can be taken orally by prescription from doctors, if they determine that you have a sufficiently severe case of adrenal deficiency to warrant oral steroids.

President John Kennedy qualified for this treatment when he was treated for Addison's Disease. You may not have Addison's, but you might indeed benefit from some of the medicine he found so helpful.

Most people do not have a severe amount of adrenal insufficiency. Their adrenal glands are nevertheless unable to make the right amount of cortisol, even with the proper vitamins, herbs, and precursors. When this is the prevailing situation, the addition of bioidentical hydrocortisone in very small amounts is sometimes miraculously beneficial. It is best used for short-term therapy, measured in weeks.

Hydrocortisone is a steroid, as are all your sex hormones, such as testosterone and estrogen. So is aldosterone, which controls your kidney function, water retention, and blood pressure. Steroids are not inherently bad substances. Everyone's body uses steroids every day, and we need them. It is part of our normal metabolism. If you are still too low in adrenal power, no matter how hard you try to balance things, then you may want to try a brief course of low-dose prescription hydrocortisone. Note that we're talking about *natural cortisone*. The natural bioidentical forms of the hormones are quite important, as you may have seen in our last chapter on reproductive system balance.

There are many types of cortisone *not* to use. These include all the synthetic cortisones that are commonly available and widely used for severe illness. A person who is prescribed powerful synthetic prednisone for severe asthma or terrible rheumatoid arthritis often finds the medicine very helpful for these severe illnesses when used carefully. A person who needs some mild adrenal balancing should *not* use synthetic prednisone, but instead needs natural hydrocortisone. The synthetic hormones can be ten to twenty times stronger than their bioidentical counterparts, and they have very different effects on the body. Once it is established that you might benefit from a trial of bioidentical hydrocortisone, the most sensible course of action is to start at a *very* small amount and taper upward incrementally, and only as needed.

A small amount of hydrocortisone is 5 mg, the smallest pill commercially made. We recommend that you start with *half* of such a pill, once a day in the morning with breakfast. Always take your hydrocortisone with a meal, or good-size snack. If after several days you are tolerating this dose, and having a fine result, then just stick with it for a month or two, and then go off the medicine by reversing the tapering process.

If, however, you do not notice much benefit at one half of a 5 mg pill, then you may have started too low. Try increasing to a slightly higher amount. This might mean taking one whole pill daily in the morning with breakfast. Do this for five or six days to see what kind of benefit, if any, you receive. When you are low in cortisone, and you take some, the benefits are usually noticed quickly. If you do fine on that dose, then you can continue at this level for a few weeks, letting your body adjust to the improvement.

If, on the other hand, this has not been helpful, then consider trying slightly more. Keep taking the 5 mg pill in the morning with breakfast, but now add half a pill with lunch. Do this for about a week as well. By the time you have taken one whole pill with breakfast and one whole pill with lunch, you should see some improvement if low cortisol was your problem.

If you are somewhat better, you may eventually want to work your way up to the Dr. William Jeffries's protocol dose of 5 mg with breakfast, lunch, dinner, and bedtime snack. This amounts to 20 mg a day, which you could continue for five or six weeks before slowly tapering down to no prescription medicine once again. (This is more fully explained by endocrinology professor Jeffries in his classic book *Safe Uses of Cortisone*—see page 265 at the end of this book.)

During the five or six weeks of this trial, your adrenal gland may experience a rest, and therefore derive some needed healing. Now you can enjoy the beneficial results that accompany a more normalized adrenal function, even as you totally taper off the prescription medicine.

On the other hand, if 5 mg four times daily was of little to no benefit, then you and your practitioner might conclude that cortisone therapy was not for you. It might now be time to seek another approach.

This same tapering up and then tapering down method can be utilized with other forms of prescription adrenal support. A common version of this, preferred by many practitioners, is **liquid prescription adrenal-cortex drops.** Have your practitioner order from a compounding pharmacy the prescription drops in a potency equivalent to 1 drop = 1 mg of hydrocortisone.

In this way, you can perform the tapering maneuver described above with 5 drops in the morning with breakfast, instead of a 5 mg commercially made pill. The rest of the protocol for the pills is also similar for the drops.

Regardless of whether you use drops or pills, to increase the chances that the more normalized adrenal function you derive while on the prescription medication will continue once you stop taking the medicine, always combine the prescription with the natural protocols mentioned earlier. These over-the-counter agents help with the actual improvement and healing of the gland in ways that cortisol or other chemical medicines cannot.

The best use of cortisone is as a temporary assist in running your metabolic engine, while the adrenal gland has an opportunity to recuperate and heal. Sometimes the addition of cortisone is necessary initially to get other tissues functioning a little more normally, so that several organs can derive some of the healing they need as well. In these cases, prescription hydrocortisone is part of a larger program of multigland restoration, rather than just providing adrenal balancing. We heartily recommend it for this purpose, as well.

Now that you have tried your own best mix of natural and prescription medicine, perhaps your adrenal system is functioning more smoothly. How long do you continue the over-the-counter support maneuvers?

Their use is generally measured not in weeks or months, but in seasons of the year. Eventually, however, you may taper off from the over-the-counter rebalancing agents, and enjoy having your system purring along smoothly on its own.

THE BENEFITS OF ADRENAL BALANCE

Once you have accomplished some successful intervention with natural protocols, or perhaps with prescription added, then you are in a position to reap the rewards. There are great benefits that can arise from adrenal balance. An **emotional** endo-type can look forward to improvement on a variety of fronts.

Since the *adrenal gland regulates the sodium and potassium levels* in the body, a rebalanced adrenal metabolism will feel much more comfortable. Sodium and potassium are the key constituents that help differentiate between the intracellular environment (cell cytoplasm, where some chemicals are broken down and new chemicals are made) and the extracellular fluid (bloodstream, where these components are carried from organ to organ along the great river of blood vessels).

In addition, the blood pressure is now under better control, due to improved kidney function and water balance. Now you will also have the benefit of proper inflammatory response. With abnormal cortisol function, you don't fight infection or inflammation nearly as well as you would with normal amounts. Optimal levels help regulate white blood cells, especially the lymphocytes, which manage immune function.

One of the more important benefits of rebalanced adrenal hormones is that now you have more proper amounts of glucocorticoids. These help to regulate blood glucose and prevent diabetes, prediabetes, hypoglycemia, and the insulin resistance of syndrome X. This syndrome is a collection of symptoms consisting of high blood pressure, central obesity, polycystic ovaries, and a decreased sensitivity to the effects of insulin.

Who would have guessed that better balance of the adrenal glands results in a much better balance of all these sugar-regulatory mechanisms? The result is that you are no longer battling hypoglycemia. You can now have a morning breakfast, perhaps then a midmorning snack, a normal lunch, without suffering the highs and lows of fluctuating blood sugar so common to the **emotional** endo-types. You can have normal energy for the entire day without feeling that you are at the mercy of whatever it is you are eating.

Better cortisol levels also result in more balanced electrical activity of the brain. Specifically, there is a much more normalized sleep pattern and for some people fewer asthma attacks. Previously, there might have been too little cortisol in the morning and too much in the evening, resulting in the night owl syndrome. Now, insomnia and erratic sleep patterns are a thing of the past. They become normalized when the adrenal becomes balanced, allowing you to progress from being a person who finds it unbearably hard to get up in the morning to one who pops up easily when the alarm rings.

You now have a more normal emotional balance; you can respond appropriately and have various feelings without being "blown out" by them. Moreover, you have the grace and calm to go through life without feeling like a leaf blown around by every breeze that comes along.

A car can backfire, and it doesn't rattle you. An obnoxious driver may cut you off at an intersection, but you no longer fret or fume for a while afterward. Your boss can tell you about something that you need to improve on, and it doesn't demoralize you for the rest of the day, or week. You feel more solid and steady. You have more resistance to the stressors of life. You are a stronger, more resilient person.

LEARN HOW ADRENAL BALANCE AFFECTS THYROID AND SEX-HORMONE BALANCE

Now that your adrenal function is better, your thyroid might be working better, as well. Recall from our earlier discussion about how the conversion from transport thyroid hormone (T4) into active thyroid hormone (T3) requires the right amount of adrenal hormone. Too much or too little cortisol interferes with that important conversion. Now that you are more balanced, you are likely to have *more normal amounts of*

T3. Your *weight, skin, hair, and temperature regulation* may be more normal, too.

Another benefit is *less thyroid inflammation*, because the adrenal balance has helped with inflammatory improvement all over your body.
With less thyroiditis, you not only have better thyroid function, but you
also have less autoimmune response. Now you have handled one of the
major underlying difficulties, thus balancing your adrenal really does affect your thyroid for the better.

Beyond whatever additional thyroid health you attain from enhanced
adrenal balance, there is also *adrenal benefit for your reproductive system*. A
healthy adrenal makes plenty of sex hormones. In males, the adrenal gland
is the only source of estrogen and progesterone, which men absolutely
need. In females, the adrenal gland is the only source of testosterone,
which women absolutely need. You can see that your adrenal glands are
necessary for a complete complement of reproductive hormones.

Therefore, when the adrenal is functioning well, you are more likely
to have the *right sex-hormone balance*. For women, the end result is less
PMS, and more normal periods. For older women, it means a more
comfortable menopause.

If you are male, you now have greater balance between your as-
sertiveness and your sensitivity. You might be less prone to excess stomach acid and to general worry and concern. Your digestion might be
better, maybe with fewer headaches and less tight muscles.

Both sexes might notice an *increase in libido*. One of the less understood reasons for low sex drive in both men and women is abnormal
adrenal activity. If you are frequently dealing with "fight or flight" feelings, you don't have much energy left over for amorous thoughts or acts.
If you are constantly feeling challenged, existing in survival mode, that
leaves little space for expressions of love or sexual desire.

It should be very clear by now that a surprising amount of life and
health is controlled by our adrenal glands. They play a major part in our
basic function in the world.

When you are an **emotional** endo-type and you rebalance your adrenals, you frequently have what amounts to a totally new life. You are now
a more comfortable, centered, and congenial person. You move through

life with greater equanimity, courage, and focus. There is no setting of a price tag on this kind of benefit. It is worth more than gold itself.

CONCEPT SUMMARY

1. We encourage you to work with your practitioner to make this rebalancing effort a very creative and self-driven process, an honest reflection of *your* own beliefs, visions, and inner guidance.
2. The adrenal gland has a very peculiar way of slowing down when it has been overtaxed. It fails in the manner of a large dying star, which gets brighter and brighter before it burns out.
3. Selye defined *stress* as "general adaptation syndrome." He identified three phases: (1) alarm (2) adaptation, (3) exhaustion.
4. Without diagnosis and treatment, adrenal insufficiency can create havoc in your life. It is difficult to evaluate properly because there are several stages of insufficiency.
5. Often, adrenal imbalance requires the help of a high-level practitioner, though occasionally it can be managed on one's own. If you are an **emotional** endo-type, based upon self-evaluations and home tests, you might initiate some of the simplest adrenal rebalancing steps by yourself and see how it goes. Adrenal is one gland that, when altered, can make you quickly feel either really good, or truly miserable. Fortunately, small corrections can create fast and welcome relief.

ACTION SUMMARY

❑ The **emotional** endo-type should move toward a carefully balanced, middle-of-the road eating plan that includes high-quality food taken in small frequent meals.

❑ Extra salt can be good for **emotional** endo-types, especially if you have had low blood pressure. For those with possible thyroid involvement, you might try sea salt or noniodized salt, and check your blood pressure weekly.

❑ Avoid CATS (caffeine, alcohol, tobacco, sugar—and we also recommend avoiding chocolate). These give temporary boosts and leave you feeling exhausted and craving more of them.

*There are certain vitamins and minerals that help **emotional** endo-types:*

❑ Pantothenic acid (B₅). 250 mg 2 to 3 times daily

❑ Vitamin B₆. 50 mg 2 to 3 times daily

❑ Phosphorylated Serine—brand name SeriPhos (not phosphatidyl serine)—is quite handy if you take 1,000 mg one hour prior to a high cortisol time of day, as measured by your saliva test. (Good for Stage II adrenal problems in general and especially good for sleep when taken at bedtime.)

❑ Full-strength licorice (not the deglycerized DLG type). 300 mg tablet daily for the first week, increase by one tablet of 300 mg daily for each of the next several weeks (second week take two tablets daily, third week take three tablets daily); be sure to check blood pressure weekly

Add tonifying/adaptogenic herbs if needed:

❑ Ashwagandha root powder. 600 mg per day

❑ Asian ginseng (*Panax*). 400 mg daily of a root extract, standardized to 8 percent ginsenosides

❑ Cordyceps. 800 mg daily, cordicepic acid standardized 8 percent extract

❑ Rhodiola root extract. 100 mg daily standardized to 1 percent salidroside

❑ Bacopa. 500 mg daily of a leaf extract standardized to 16 percent bacosides

Then try precursor augmentation:

❑ DHEA. daily dose 5 to 10 mg with upward titration very gently to practitioner-supervised upper limits of 25 to 50 mg daily

❑ Pregnenolone. 50 to 100 mg daily

Then use *natural adrenal gland substance* (desiccated gland)—start with one pill every other day, progress gradually to one per day, then increase by another per day to three to four per day over a number of weeks.

❑ One version of this is the high-quality product IsoCort, a highly purified adrenal glandular.

❑ Another way is to use adrenal glandular liquid, sold in dropper bottles at health food stores. A stronger version of this is sold by compounding pharmacies, available by prescription.

❑ A third way would be to use homeopathic adrenal. Usually the 3x or 6x potency is utilized, and 3 pellets are dissolved under the tongue three times daily for three weeks.

Get further testing if needed:

❑ Twenty-four-hour urine sample to measure cortisol and DHEA. (You can also get a blood sample for cortisol and DHEA-S.) Insist on a free and total cortisol, with DHEA-S (DHEA sulfate). Be sure the blood specimens are collected at 8 a.m. and 4 p.m.

❑ Twenty-four-hour urine or one-time blood sample for catecholamines

❑ ACTH measurement, also ACTH stimulation test.

❑ If further help is needed, consider the addition of prescription bioactive *hydrocortisone*. Use only natural bioidentical hormone. Start with very small amounts, half of a 5 mg pill, for the first several days or week. Always take your hydrocortisone with a meal. If you do well, stay on that dose. If not, continue to add 1 or 2 more pills daily over a few weeks and see if that helps. If you reach 10 mg and still are not feeling at all improved, cortisone is probably not your medicine of choice. This is a short-term therapy, and it should be discontinued after a number of weeks.

❑ You can also try liquid prescription adrenal-cortex drops. Have your practitioner order from a compounding pharmacy that can prepare the prescription drops in a potency equivalent to 1 drop = 1 mg of hydrocortisone. Then use the same dose protocol as with the pills.

There are multiple advantages to this adrenal balancing:

- adrenal gland regulates the sodium and potassium levels
- optimal kidney function and water balance
- proper inflammatory response
- glucocorticoids to help regulate blood glucose

- helps regulate sleep patterns
- better emotional balance
- more normal T3 (weight, hair, skin, and temperature better)
- less thyroid inflammation
- better reproductive hormone balance (increased libido)

STEP III

SUSTAINING LONG-TERM SUCCESS

INTRODUCTION TO STEP III

We hope that by this time you are feeling noticeably better. Using this new strength, you can now initiate activities to help maintain your momentum. This final section gives you the long-term road map.

Now that you have adjusted and restored your glands, you will find activities here to help you keep your reclaimed endo-balance forever. Each individual endo-type is given specific attention, so that you might sustain your highest health for years to come.

For this final step of the program, we recommend that you pace yourself appropriately. Add long-term tools gradually, comfortably, and in the order that makes the most sense *for you*!

Finally, we urge you to approach these challenges philosophically and with good humor. Learn to be gentle with yourself and to give more generously to yourself. You deserve to have, and honor, your own personal program and timing as you move toward looking and feeling your best.

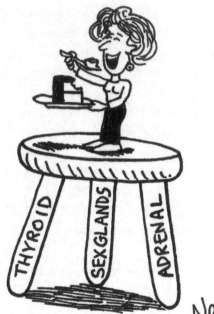

CHAPTER 9

LOOK AND FEEL YOUR BEST
MAINTAIN A COMFORTABLE BODY WEIGHT, ENERGY LEVEL, AND OUTLOOK

... to eat, and to drink, and to be merry.

—Ecclesiastes

Phoebe, as you now know, had been overweight most of her life. Once she normalized her thyroid hormone levels, her story changed. She was finally able to lose some of her excess weight and to keep the weight off, using over-the-counter thyroid interventions coupled with managing her diet and maintaining a healthy exercise program.

With the addition of proper nutrients, exercise, stress reduction maneuvers, and self-care, all targeted for her specific endo-type, she appears glowing and self-confident. She is rarely depressed these days. Menopause has come and gone. Phoebe is now comfortably postmenopausal, having sailed through this change with greater ease and comfort than the experiences of her late forties would have suggested.

While it may seem like a lot of effort to the beginner, starting simply and adding new steps regularly can become a comfortable way of life that can be easily sustained in the long run. Rather than temporary fixes, Phoebe's program is an ongoing practice that keeps her strong, happy, and healthy, regardless of the underlying tendencies that previously ruled her life. Not only does she enjoy taking care of herself, but this plan has also contributed to very positive developments in her work and family life.

LONG-TERM CHALLENGES OF THE THYROID-DRIVEN ENDO-TYPE

Some of the steps taken to jump-start your thyroid should not be continued indefinitely, while some can be continued long-term. Our goal in this chapter is to help you ascertain which of the earlier suggestions should be continued, which should be modified, and which are no longer appropriate for you. Armed with this information, you can be aware of your tendencies and keep them in check. The idea is simply to live a full and balanced life, honoring your body and its unique needs.

But first, let's identify the long-term challenges for people with compromised thyroid function.

Weight Problems

If you are like many other thyroid-driven endo-types, most likely you have already tried a number of diets. Thyroid-challenged people need to understand that for them, the simple maneuver of eating fewer calories and getting more exercise does not exactly apply. You might make no progress at all, despite heroic efforts, if your energy hormones are out of balance.

You may know some folks who are as thin as a rail, who can eat as much as they want and don't gain weight. Other people can eat one muffin and put on three pounds! We think this has something to do with the amount of the thyroid hormone you have available, and how well it is working.

Whether or not you derive a lot of useful energy and heat from your food, or simply store excess weight, might well be related to your metabolism, a topic which is still not completely understood by medical science. Each person needs to consider his or her food intake and pay attention to the body's response to various food items.

The Depression Connection to Weight

Depression is the mental expression of exhaustion, which can happen physically through depletion of neurotransmitters, the chemicals that transmit energy along the pathways of the nervous system. For many of us, this continuous flow of neurochemicals has been altered. The confusion generated through competition on receptor sites can cause flooding of certain chemicals, and a reduction in others.

For reasons mentioned earlier, many people today are feeling depressed, especially as they age. There can, of course, be other reasons for lowered biochemicals. One of these, as we've mentioned many times, is the epidemic of low thyroid, underpowering our glands and thereby resulting in depletion of many necessary body chemicals.

Energy: Having the Steam to Live Out Your Dream!

Few things in life are as frustrating—or depressing—as knowing what you *want* to do, but not having the energy to accomplish it. Though low energy can result from a great variety of conditions, it is a classic and almost universal symptom of slow metabolic function.

In fact, energy, weight, and depression are closely related. When people carry excess weight, it is often difficult for them to feel energetic. This causes them to move less and gain more weight, and to feel worse about it all the while. When they are finally able to lose some of the excess weight, they find themselves feeling lighter, more active, and eager to accomplish their goals. Excess weight can also result in lowered self-esteem, making it increasingly challenging for the person to strive toward her dreams. In fact, these folks often become depressed and inactive, losing sight of their purpose and goals.

As Phoebe, our **physical** endo-type friend from chapter 1, embarked upon her healing program, she realized that she would have to make many changes, on different levels, in order to feel better. She followed our "thyroid driven endo-type energy conservation recommendations" which included

- creating a circle of support
- selecting practitioners who listened carefully to her
- learning to screen people as to whether they enhanced or drained her when she was around them
- learning to assert herself to enhance her energy flow

Some people find that in combatting subtle energy flow challenges, improving mental concepts (thoughts) can prove highly beneficial. That may mean temporarily seeing a counselor or therapist, to determine the roots of unhealthy thinking, and to replace those patterns with more positive ones.

For others, this may mean adding daily meditation, relaxation, or the use of affirmations—positive statements considered by some to be "food for the soul." An example might be "I feel peaceful and calm" when agitated, or "My body responds easily and effortlessly to exercise." Positive thoughts change the chemicals in our brain in a way that causes a different response in our physical body. As the renowned "sleeping prophet" Edgar Cayce, considered to be America's foremost psychic, once said in his readings ". . . For the spirit is life; the mind is the builder; the physical is the result." (Edgar Cayce readings, number 349–4)

Our emotions are a very valuable feedback mechanism, not to be ignored. They often tell us what we need to do in order to live more comfortably and what we need to pay attention to in our lives. After experiencing emotional situations, you may find that certain memories or feelings resurface regularly or occasionally. Each time this happens, you are given another opportunity to heal the memory or experience. When we have deeply disturbing events occur, it can take many years to process the memories and release the pain associated with them. This kind of emotional release work must be dealt with in a very safe environment, with highly trained professionals.

Emotional baggage can be a major energy drain. For those who are energetically compromised, dealing with past hurts and learning to work with love and forgiveness can be astoundingly healing. This means that if you were abused as a child, emotionally, physically, sexually, or in other ways, you will at some point need to find ways to release the trauma associated with this.

For many people, this frequently means working with a trained therapist. It can involve talking, crying, raging, shaking, writing, movement, or using other creative methods to release the actual stress from your physical body. Remember the body is like a road map of your life. How we walk, talk, think, and look often relate to the experiences we've had in our lives. Ultimately, these can shape how we appear to the world, how we carry ourselves, even how our facial features look.

Our mission is not just to repair tired glands, but also to restore our multidimensional wholeness. The sense of loss and despair mentioned in the preface of this book can permeate our beings on every level—physically, mentally, emotionally and spiritually. We must fight back with tools on each level for complete restoration of health.

In recent years, various forms of healing have arisen that can be helpful in restoring wholeness. Try to include creative movement, body-work, or other therapies to supplement your healing program. Allow your creativity to begin to flow, and invite excellent therapists to introduce you to their tools. You will discover, as we have, the exciting and energizing wide world of healing. And through these modalities and gifted practitioners, you will find your way back to a true and lasting health, a balance that can be yours for the rest of your life.

OPTIMAL APPROACHES FOR LONG-TERM SUCCESS

We have already shared many ideas for nutritional interventions for the **physical** endo-type. They range from taking general multivitamin/multimineral combination products, adding essential fatty acids and amino acids, and eating a higher-fiber, lower-calorie diet initially to specific herbal preparations, enzymes, and natural or prescription thyroid hormone to help restore your optimal health.

**The goal for inspiring long-term health is to change
old patterns *into* more health-enhancing behaviors.**

The suggestions that we make in this chapter are specially designed to achieve a lasting rebalance, rather than backsliding into the typical New Year's resolution syndrome.

WHAT TO CONTINUE

People with sluggish metabolism need a particular complement of vitamins, minerals, and other items to sustain them for the long haul. Continue to cover the nutritional bases with the following:

Nutrients

- A good multivitamin/mineral combination (explained in chapter 5).
- The full symphony mixed antioxidant started in chapter 5.
- Magnesium. Keep in mind that there are several types of magnesium; experiment to find out which type works best for your body. Many people prefer magnesium citrate, although the gluconate is popular, as well. Both of these are generally more effective and better tolerated than magnesium oxide, so be sure to read the bottle carefully.

Glandulars

Experts differ on their degree of comfort with this particular form of therapy. At our clinic, however, we have consistently found it helpful for **physical** endo-types to take one or two pills a day of a high-quality thyroid glandular product for long-term maintenance. This is especially true if you are not taking prescription thyroid medicine. But even if you are on medication such as Synthroid or Levoxyl, it is still a worthwhile idea. (The thyroid glandulars, as mentioned previously, are made of freeze-dried thyroid gland from animals, generally pigs. This is the same source as is used for prescription dessicated thyroid, such as Armour. They help by providing additional important building blocks for thyroid metabolism).

Fun and Enjoyable Exercise for Health Maintenance

We remind you to engage in slow repetitive rhythmic exercise (to stoke your furnace without exhausting it). This can include walking, gentle bike-riding, or easygoing swimming. (Be sure to wash off thoroughly after swimming in a pool to reduce the impact of chlorine or other chemical stressors.)

In addition to exercise, and equally important, take time regularly to stretch. This can be a comfortable and slow, open-ended gentle stretching. (Recall that your muscles and tendons may not repair as quickly or as well as you'd prefer, so it's better not to push.)

Herbal Medicines

In addition to the above nutritional supplements that are helpful for long-term thyroid success, two herbal remedies can serve you nicely for the long run, regardless of what kind of thyroid medication you may have needed to reestablish balance.

The first is the ayurvedic herb ashwagandha (Latin name *Withania somnifera*), which boosts the conversion of T4 into active T3 hormone. This can be extremely valuable to those who are taking only thyroxine (T4) as their thyroid medicine. (Thyroxine is marketed as Synthroid, Levoxyl, Levothroid, Unithroid, Levo-thyroxine, and L-thyroxine.) Those taking T3 hormone (Cytomel) should also try ashwagandha, which may result in less T3 medication needed.

Try Asian ginseng (*Panax*), for its stimulant and adaptogenic properties. Recall that the adaptogens are chemicals that help a hormone to be more balanced at its binding site. Therefore, if you have not been taking ashwagandha or ginseng up to this point, you may want to experiment with them, one at a time, to see if they help you to feel even more restored and balanced. For the long haul, these adaptogenic herbs can be highly helpful.

WHAT TO ADD TO YOUR PROGRAM

Better Drinking Water

In addition to toxins building up in the fat of animals, a great many toxins are inadvertently building up in and sometimes deliberately being added to the water available for us to drink. As this now serious problem worsens, you can protect yourself by filtering your drinking water. A good carbon-block filter will remove most of the impurities, organisms, and heavy metals. (See page 272 for specific information on water filtration devices.) Don't assume that the costly bottled water that seems to be so pristine is any better than tap water. This industry is not highly regulated. Water filtration devices also vary enormously in their ability to protect you. For a list of companies and products that are certified, consult the Web site for the National Sanitation Foundation (www.nsf.org).

Better than these above choices would be water derived *from reverse osmosis filtration*, as is sold in bulk in various grocery and health food stores. These units can also be purchased and used at home. Ideally your water would be free from chlorine, bromine, fluorine, as well as contaminants.

Additional Antioxidants

Here are some specific additional antioxidants for long-term use:

- Quercetin 500 mg daily
- Pygnogenol 150 mg daily

These antioxidants fight free radicals in your system, which are the result of oxidative stress. Our cells and tissues are continuously subjected to highly reactive molecules known as free radicals, the harmful by-products of cellular metabolism, as well as byproducts of an industrial society. They undermine our health when their numbers increase to a point of harmful accumulation, which is what is meant by "oxidative stress."

This situation, unchallenged, can lead to cell damage and cell death. The *antioxidants help to clear these damaging substances* that can make us feel tired or sick. Some vitamins act as antioxidants by helping to clear free radicals; other nutrients help us by supporting the overall detoxification processes that occur largely in the liver.

Energy Conservation

If you are energy-compromised, what can you do to make better use of the energy you have? Pay attention to your energy level. When is it up? When is it down? What seems to be causing the fluctuations? Is there a rhythm in your energy flow? If so, try to chart that over a twenty-four-hour period noting the time of food, drink, and activity.

This kind of attention to detail will benefit you greatly as you move into a larger role of self-advocacy and guidance. Watching, perhaps first as an objective observer, the ups and downs of your energy flow will enable you to come to grips with where you are gaining energy and, perhaps most important for the energy-compromised person, where you are losing energy. Some of these revelations might be quite surprising!

If there are certain times of the day that you feel consistently drained or depleted, you may need to augment with specific nutrients and foods in order to avoid these disruptive variations.

Stress Reduction

We strongly encourage you to make this a critical piece of your ongoing program. The **physical** endo-type benefits well from stress reduction and meditative techniques that are unstructured. You might simply think of a comfortable vacation you've taken in the past, or one you've imagined in your mind's eye. Focus on the various aspects that made it so enjoyable. If you notice your mind wandering to more stressful thoughts, gently refocus on the vacation, and pull the mind back. Deep breathing can be extremely relaxing, as well as restorative to your energy, and it can be coupled with quiet reflective time taken daily to release tension.

Bodywork

At this stage of maintenance for your reclaimed health, consider adding some bodywork. This might involve seeking Swedish massage, which provides a slow, comfortable touch. If you enjoy and tolerate bodywork well, you might also possibly add some lymphatic flow massage, which gently assists the flow of lymphatic drainage as it moves through the body.

Gentle Jumping

Also remember that our lymph system, which helps to escort toxins out, does not have its own pump! It relies on some bouncy activity on your part, whether this is accomplished through your brisk walks or other methods. Many people enjoy jumping gently on a bouncer, which looks like a small trampoline. It can help you pump your lymph, using gentle or more vigorous movement, all the while protecting your spine and knees from impact injury. On page 272 we have listed the name of a company that makes a very sturdy jumper for personal use (and folds in half and can be put under a bed or out of sight easily).

Hypnosis

This can be quite successful in helping a thyroid-challenged person to lose weight. There are people who have been able to turn their lack of success around with the use of hypnosis, sometimes losing fifty, seventy-five, or one hundred pounds. These people may have had internal psychological drive for overeating or internal chemistry that selectively stored fat. The hypnotic state allows for internal rebalancing homeostasis to take hold. Your inner drive to a better equilibrium may be augmented by visualizing your restorative systems stabilizing the three energy hormones.

Acupuncture

For thyroid, there is hardly anything better than the health enhancement provided by acupuncture. The subtle energies that can be aligned and directed by focus on meridian boosting and balance seem to have a marvelous salutary effect on thyroid tissue and overall thyroid metabolism.

Aromas

To your ongoing program for health maintenance, you might explore the gentle art of aromatherapy. Thyroid-driven types are often tired, so the stimulating use of *myrtle*, or *mint scented essential oils*, can provide the boost you need to get through the day and help restore your glands.

Colors

In addition to smells, which stimulate the brain in a particular way to enhance vital activity, you can also have fun learning more about color therapy, which significantly affects mood and energy. Very helpful for your situation might be the color *blue*, which is the color associated with the throat energy center (fifth chakra). It is often used in healing throat or thyroid issues.

Flower Remedies

For those who want to work with very gentle tools to stimulate their own healing, you might add certain well-chosen flower remedies. These are made from the oils of specific flowers, and have been used by many cultures for health promotion. The best known are the *Bach flower remedies*, created by Dr. Edward Bach in the 1930s. There are also several companies in California and elsewhere that make lovely flower remedies. These remedies seem to work largely on the mental plane, but can be a very helpful adjunct to the other therapies listed here.

For the person who is tired, you may consider the flower remedy *gorse* (when long-term illness causes one to lose faith in the healing ability), or *olive* (drained of energy, exhausted). In a different company's system (North American Flower Essences made in Nevada City, California), a likely choice for the **physical** endo-type might be *California pitcher plant* or *Indian paintbrush*.

Lastly, here is one final item you might add to your program. In consideration of your tendency to feel depleted and perhaps down, we highly recommend that you include as much unstructured time as possible in your life. Many people feel rejuvenated when they relax, so scheduling yourself tightly most of the time will have the opposite effect of what your system needs. To the extent that you can choose your schedule, arrange for more free time whenever possible.

WHAT TO AVOID

Just as there are many items listed above for you to take, there are also some very important things you need to avoid for the long-term health you seek.

Bad Fats

The worst choices of all are the trans-fats, also known as partially hydrogenated oils. This especially means to avoid such hard fats as Crisco. Consider margarine, touted as the ideal "butter" substitute. For years, margarine has been considered an improvement over the solid animal fat of cream on the top of milk, which gets churned into butter. The problem with margarine is that to form it into a stick, the fats need to be hardened or hydrogenated, so they will maintain a more solid state at room temperature. We recommend avoiding this food. The tub forms of margarine seem better because they are softer, but many of them are still partially hydrogenated. Trans-fats interfere with our normal lipid metabolism, apparently increasing the deposit of plaque in our arteries and fat on our bodies.

Pesticides in Foods, Hormones in Meats

Remember that toxins store in the fat of animals, so less fatty and organically raised animals are your best bet. Mainly, keep in mind from our discussion in chapter 2 that to ingest less of these toxic pollutants, you may need to ingest as little animal fat as you comfortably can. The red meats have the highest fat content, particularly marbled beef or fatty hamburger.

Foods That Don't Agree with You

This broad category addresses the well-known fact that each of us has *specific sensitivities and allergies* that we must pay attention to, or pay the price. There are medical clinics that test for delayed food sensitivities, helping you to know which items are causing which problems in your body systems.

Chlorides, Fluorides, and Bromides in Air, Food, Water

These halogens tend to bind on the receptor sites where your thyroid hormone might need to be in order to keep things moving properly. Do your best to continue the process of replacing chlorinated household chemicals with more natural ones from the health food store, that are biodegradable and nontoxic.

Iodine—Friend or Foe?

As mentioned in chapter 6, while iodine is another halogen from the same family as chlorine and bromine, this topic is important enough to warrant its own category. Iodine is essential to the production of your two key thyroid hormones (T3 and T4). What is really important for you to understand is that a significant percentage of people with autoimmune thyroid disease are *very* sensitive to iodine, and increased exposure can aggravate their situation and make their symptoms worse. There are current efforts under way to find better methods to evaluate iodine status. While we are following these developments carefully, we have yet to be convinced that specific additional iodine supplementation is a good idea for people with autoimmune thyroid disorders. Stay in touch with our website, and other thyroid-related sites that discuss research developments, and we will attempt to keep readers informed over time. For long-term health if you have a thyroid issue, we recommend against using more iodine than is in foods or regular vitamin products.

Goitrogens (Foods That Cause Goiters)

This category of food substances includes sorghum, walnuts, peanuts, pine nuts, millet, tapioca, soy products, broccoli, brussel sprouts, cabbage, cauliflower, turnip, mustard greens, spinach, rutabaga, and aspartame. We are not saying you must avoid these items, but rather that you might continue your improvement by not overindulging in them. Particularly surprising to many health-oriented people is the large category of *soy*, from which soy milk, soy cheeses, soybeans and nuts, soy powders, and many other products derive. While soy is touted as an excellent food containing phytoestrogens (plant forms of estrogen), and is therefore often recommended for midlife women, it also has a downside for autoimmune thyroid types.

One key component of soy, the isoflavones, can trigger or worsen a thyroid condition. Specifically, genistin demonstrates toxicity in the thyroid by inhibiting peroxidase, one of the enzymes needed to help assemble T4. Especially avoid highly concentrated forms of soy, such as soy powders.

"Toxic" Work Environment

Many workplace environments are created using chemical-laden products that can affect sensitive people quite negatively. In addition to the toxins, they frequently rely upon air-conditioned recycled air, without access to "clean air" (fresh air) from the outside. Artificial lighting can be stressful for sensitive people, as can other chemical cleaners used in the work environment. While we cannot always control every aspect of our workplace, we certainly can make efforts to minimize the harmful aspects of products being used in our environments by becoming vocal (join a committee), or, if you work in a large company, exerting pressure for healthier accommodations.

Similarly, if you feel that you work in an emotionally unhealthy environment, do what you can to minimize your stress, learning to guard your energy and keeping things in perspective. Keep breathing, and use some of your newfound relaxation tools to maintain balance.

"Toxic" Home Environment

Also, if you are living in a stressful home environment, now would be an excellent time for you to begin to tackle things that you can change. There are dozens of books about how to improve your environment, minimizing the chemical exposures that can be avoided, and minimizing the stressful emotional encounters that may be draining your much-needed energy, some of which we have recommended in Further Reading.

False Weight-Loss Products

You may be bombarded by advertising for common "nutritional weight-loss products" that may not be in your best interests. There are too many to mention them all, but here are our opinions on some of the most popular but ill-advised "weight-reduction" and "energy-boosting" products:

>   *Chromium:* Available in a variety of forms at vitamin stores, chromium is indeed an important mineral that might be helpful in regulating blood sugar, but it might not be helpful for weight loss by itself. It may reduce sweet cravings or help to stabilize glucose levels somewhat, but is not really a weight-loss product.
>
>   *Carnitine:* Sometimes called l-carnitine, this is an amino acid that is supposed to help people lose weight by increasing energy and

muscle mass. No one amino acid will do that alone. It has been a useful nutrient, but is not the answer for weight problems, except perhaps for a few people with unusually low levels to start with.

CLA (conjugated linoleic acid): A very popular product reputed to speed up metabolism and increase muscle size, but has not been shown to be an effective solo remedy for weight loss.

Pyruvate or pyruvic acid: Another item commonly sold in drug stores, health food stores, and multilevel companies. Our bodies normally utilize this in metabolizing carbohydrates; some had claimed it was a wonderful way to lose weight without even trying, but so far it hasn't been shown to be effective as was promised. Originally thought to be a breakthrough, it now looks more like a dud!

Phenylpropanolamine: Used in cold remedies and antihistamine combinations and weight-reduction tablets (Dexatrim, Accutrim), this was banned a few years ago. Like the previously banned "phen-fen," it had too many side effects and, while sometimes effective for the short term, it was also harmful in the long run.

Herbs: Herbs sold for weight loss are generally herbal diuretics, not actual adipose tissue reducers. They can help with water retention and high blood pressure for those who don't want to use prescription medicines, but in the end don't really help you to lose weight. Examples of *diuretic herbs* are dandelion, cleavers, cornsick, oatstraw, asparagus, hawthorne, juniper, horsetail, and shadegrass. Continuous use of these could result in excessive loss of sodium or potassium, which are crucial body salts.

Fiber: Used to make one feel full and thereby eat less, fiber can be useful for cleansing and keeping up good bowel flow. It can also help lower cholesterol by aiding its excretion from the GI tract. Fiber is healthy and may make you feel more full, but rarely by itself will fiber help with weight loss.

One of the *worst things* you can do for weight loss is to try to lose pounds by taking natural stimulants. Often the main stimulant ingredient is caffeine. Sometimes it is ephedra, also known as ma huang, sales of which have been curtailed recently due to liver damage and other dangerous side effects. Ephedra, like ephedrine, is a powerful stimulant.

Guarana, the seeds of a plant from Brazil, is a very strong stimulant that is very high in caffeine and causes lots of side effects. Additional stimulants to avoid include cola nut, from Africa. Gotu kola is a common herb, somewhat similar, but not as strong as cola nut.

Overall, none of these natural stimulants is helpful for weight loss in the long run, and most can be addictive. Moreover, they have side effects such as insomnia, high blood pressure, dehydration, and agitation.

A ROAD MAP FOR PHYSICAL ENDO-TYPES

In order to effect healthy change in your life and continue to enhance your energy, you might need to

Invite more curiosity into your life. Rather than accepting what you are told, particularly regarding your health and medical condition, you will need to reclaim some of your childlike wonder in considering what might be true for *you.* Remember that when practitioners speak of the statistics, they are talking about averages and norms. You will need to make the decision for yourself that you are *not* a statistic, but a human person with will and choice to exert in any given situation.

Create a circle of support around you, inviting those who are positive and nourishing in your life to be a part of that circle. Be sure to choose carefully; you may love someone, but need to look at him or her objectively in terms of determining whether or not he or she is appropriate for this circle of support. Some friends make you laugh, and you enjoy being with them, but they cannot show up when needed. This person should not be included in your circle of support, which needs to involve people who *will* be there.

Improve your ability to reach out to others. Many of us have been raised to help others and not to ask for help. To reclaim more of your energy and to restore your health, you may now be in a position where you must accept support. Remember that allowing yourself to receive is as important as giving, and that to complete the flow of energy through your life, you need to allow the cycle of giving and receiving to flow through you.

CONCEPT SUMMARY

1. No one diet can be right for everyone. It is crucial that you learn to listen to your own body and make adjustments accordingly.
2. The goal for inspiring long-term health is to change old habits and patterns toward more health-enhancing behaviors.

ACTION SUMMARY

THINGS TO CONTINUE TAKING

- ❑ A good multivitamin/multimineral combination
- ❑ Full-symphony mixed antioxidant
- ❑ Magnesium (magnesium citrate, or gluconate are better tolerated than magnesium oxide)
- ❑ Glandulars (one or two pills a day of a high-quality thyroid glandular product for long-term maintenance, especially if not taking prescription thyroid medicine)
- ❑ Ashwagandha (Latin name, *Withania somnifera*), which boosts conversion of T4 into active T3 hormone and can be extremely valuable to those taking only thyroxine (T4) as their thyroid medicine
- ❑ Asian ginseng (Latin name, *Panax ginseng*), another tonifier and balancer that's very useful for general energy enhancement

WHAT TO ADD TO YOUR PROGRAM

- ❑ *Better drinking water* (reverse osmosis or carbon block filter)
- ❑ *Specific additional antioxidants*
  - ❑ Quercetin, 500 mg daily
  - ❑ Pygnogenol, 150 mg daily
- ❑ *Stress reduction*
  - ❑ Meditation (unstructured thought observation)
  - ❑ Deep breathing
  - ❑ Hypnosis (for weight loss)
- ❑ Slow repetitive rhythmic exercise, including walking, gentle bike riding, or easygoing swimming (remember to avoid or wash off chlorine when possible)

❑ Stretching—this can be comfortably slow, open-ended gentle stretching
❑ Bodywork—gentle Swedish, perhaps lymph drainage massage
❑ Gentle jumping
❑ Acupuncture
❑ Aromatherapy
❑ Myrtle and mint essential oils
❑ Colors (red = stimulating, blue = throat-healing)
❑ *Flower remedies*
   ❑ Gorse (tired, losing faith)
   ❑ Olive (drained of energy, exhausted)

THINGS TO AVOID

❑ Bad fats (hydrogenated vegetable oils, animal fats from meat)
❑ Pesticides in foods, hormones in meats
❑ Foods that don't agree with you
❑ Chlorides, fluorides, and bromides in air, food, water
❑ Iodine (while the jury is still out, we recommend caution!)
❑ Goitrogens (see full list in text)
❑ Soy (limit intake to one serving every other day)
❑ Exposure to airborn chemicals (use filters)
❑ Toxic work environment
❑ Toxic home environment
❑ False weight-loss products, especially stimulants

GENERAL SUGGESTIONS

❑ Create more unstructured time
❑ Looser schedules
❑ Be curious, reach out
❑ Create a circle of support

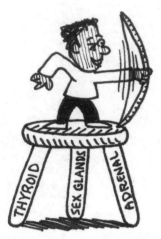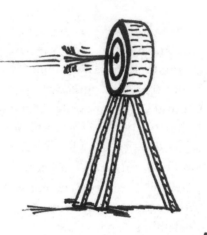

Narelle

CHAPTER 10

BE SHARP AND FOCUSED AT WORK AND PLAY
SMART NUTRIENTS PLUS MIND-POWER TECHNIQUES

> Depend upon it, sir . . . It concentrates his mind wonderfully.
>
> —Samuel Johnson

Though she had reclaimed much of her focused self, Meredith saw that she had an inner tendency to get out of focus from time to time in this new phase of her life, regardless of how much hormone cream or how many pills she used.

At one of her follow-up appointments to evaluate whether another natural remedy would be right for her, given that full-blown menopause was still to come, Meredith told us that she wanted to prepare for that stage of her life even more naturally. She saw the benefits of these natural interventions and knew there had to be something she could do besides just adding more creams and nutraceuticals to her regimen. We were all for it.

The antidote to a fuzzy-thinking hormonal life was, in Meredith's case, going to be a physical discipline. We explained to her how much more focused and clear her mind would be if she took up the practice of yoga. She laughed out loud upon hearing this suggestion. "Doc, you've got to be kidding! I'm not the yoga type! I'm a single mom with two teenaged kids, I'm the chairperson on three different school committees. I am not the type to sit on a bed of nails with my legs crossed, my head in a turban, and my mouth full of raw sunflower seeds."

We laughed and told Meredith that this was far from an accurate description of a modern yoga-class participant. In fact, it was our impression, as we related it to her, that those classes were filled with women just like her, many of whom have derived great focus and clarity from their new practice. Once Meredith understood how the focused movement and breathing—and the concentration on the sensation—would help sharpen her mind as well as forestall her family's tendency toward arthritis, she decided to give it a try. She signed up for a class at the nearby junior college and was amazed at how well she took to it. Not only was the stretching enjoyable, and relaxing, but she also really did feel more grounded, focused, and sharp.

As she became more comfortable experiencing her own body and her body's ability to focus her mind, she really relaxed into it, hardly aware of those around her. Over time, she became noticeably more calm, and yoga became an increasingly important part of her life.

LONG-TERM CHALLENGES OF THE MENTAL ENDO-TYPE

As Meredith's story illustrates, the special long-term challenge for the sex-gland endo-type is in being able to maintain focus and concentration amid the ups and downs of life, in general, and of internal chemistry, in specific. The sex hormones are often in flux more dramatically and erratically than the other hormones. That is because there are so many inner and outer influences exerted upon them.

The purpose of this chapter is to show you how to meet this special challenge with grace and balance. There are always distractions, interruptions, detours, and slippery slides along our life path. People who are thinking-challenged types easily get thrown off track by one or another of these influences. The **mental** endo-type needs some special help and some specific techniques for channeling that mental energy in a focused way for the most positive results. Otherwise, she can become scattered, amorphous, and diffuse, making her thinking filmy, wispy, and foggy.

How to Maintain Your Edge

Keeping your clarity and direction is part of the challenge, as you know, since the reproductive hormones are deeply entwined with brain function. One way to do this is to become more grounded. Grounding means getting your bearings and knowing your place in the world, right now. It means staying in touch with who you are and what you are here to accomplish—now, and in the long run. Grounding relates to remembering where you are, where you parked the car, and where your keys are.

Being grounded involves making a commitment to staying connected to yourself and those around you, having a written list of things to do, perhaps making yourself remember to bring the list with you. It means keeping track of how much time you will need to accomplish selected goals and knowing what to do next. It can mean having a calendar where you clearly record obligations for the future.

The popularity of Palm devices and organizers is a testament to how many of us need help focusing, given the complexity of modern life. It is not just the **mental** endo-types that benefit from organizing devices, but they especially need this kind of help. If you are this endo-type, you may want to explore carefully whatever organizational tools exist, taking care to choose ones that truly benefit you, rather than adding to your stress.

OPTIMAL APPROACHES FOR LONG-TERM SUCCESS

Another important aspect of the **mental** endo-type deals with the creative function of our reproductive hormones. Whether or not you have or plan to participate in making an actual human baby, creativity is one of the essential facets of living. Unless one is an independently wealthy couch potato, we are generally occupied to some degree with creating food, shelter, art, science, interpersonal relationships, music, poetry, and literature.

This is what makes life worth living, and your participation in it, as a **mental** endo-type, is crucial to your health. It is part of your purpose to exercise this creative aspect as only you can do. These dominant hormones were created for directing this creative force into the world. Thus, a big part of your ongoing long-term success revolves around providing time and energy for creative pursuits.

WHAT TO CONTINUE?

Long-Term Nutrition for the **Mental** Endo-Type

The worst thing a **mental** endo-type could do would be to focus on the light eating of just juices and salads. While this is a fine cleansing maneuver (and works well for certain types of people), it can be too loose and light for a person already tending to be somewhat amorphous. It simply does not provide dense enough intake for long-lasting stability.

There are a variety of high-protein diets currently available to choose from. Whether you choose to follow Dr. Atkins's approach, or some other version of the protein diet, keep this in mind: You are still hormonally challenged and need to avoid eating huge amounts of animal fat. This is where the endocrine monkey wrenches from pollution are concentrated.

Fish is an excellent protein alternative to red meat, and most Americans don't eat fish as often as might be helpful. Most forms of fish (such as salmon, herring, sardines, and mackerel) provide clean, lean protein and beneficial fats. These omega-3 oils and essential fatty acids (EFAs) help reduce the joint inflammation of arthritis and improve the function of insulin in hypoglycemics and diabetics. There are obviously a few things to watch out for in fish selection. (See page 210.)

In general, the EFAs from fish are beneficial for all of us in helping to reduce autoimmune effects as well as lower the risk of heart disease.

As part of a sensible approach to eating less animal fat, remember that the amino acids from beans combine with the amino acids from grains make a complete protein. You don't have to have a high-meat diet to eat a higher protein diet. It simply takes some experimenting with more grains and beans as part of your hormone-balancing efforts. If you combine seeds, nuts, and sprouts with grains, you will increase the amount of complete protein available to you. If you use avocados and eggs, or well-formulated protein powders, you can supplement comfortably.

The classic protein source among beans is the soybean. While thyroid-driven endo-types need to eat soy cautiously, **mental** endo-types don't have to worry so much about the goitrogenic effects of the isoflavone genistin. Aside from a thyroid-diminishing side effect at high levels of ingestion, soy is a very good way to ensure a high-protein diet. All beans have some protein, but soy has a superior amount of it.

In addition, the isoflavone components of soy are hormonally active, generally in a beneficial way. Many women have found a comfortable balance-enhancement effect with the addition of more soy foods into their diet during PMS and menopause.

Long-Term Supplementation for the **Mental** Endo-Type

For long-term maintenance of your hormonal balance, **mental** endo-types should explore slightly on higher doses of *vitamin E*, in addition to their regular multivitamin and mineral combo as outlined in chapter 5. This particular nutrient is helpful for PMS and for the hot flashes of menopause. For men, vitamin E is helpful for maintaining good connective tissue, and is involved in blood pressure regulation. For both sexes, the amount people take in by diet alone or with standard multivitamins is quite insufficient to tackle their needs. We are therefore recommending an extra 200 IUs each day for sex endo-types in general, and up to an extra 400 for menopausal women to eliminate hot flashes. (It's better and safer than estrogen!)

Another key vitamin is *folic acid*—absolutely fundamental for metabolism in general, and especially for balancing in **mental** endo-types. Since there are several forms of folate needed by the body, the best way to take it in is with 200 mcg of the new version called tetrahydrofolate—ask for it by name at a reputable health food or vitamin store.

Of particular importance for the sex gland endo-type is the mineral *magnesium*, which also in higher amounts ensures an increased rate of bowel flow. A great deal of PMS could be alleviated with the simple addition of an extra 400 to 800 mg of magnesium citrate daily. Try to determine your exact needs by increasing the amount that you take each day; start at 400 mg, see at what daily dose (600, 800, 1,000, 1,400 and so on) you begin to have softer stools. (A dose just below the amount that causes softer stools is called your "bowel tolerance.") Once again, we recommend a high-quality product that can be obtained via companies we have listed in the appendices, or at a reputable vitamin store.

Finally, to round out your long-term program, consider the amino acid *arginine*. It is very helpful for increasing your solid grounding, focus, and memory. It is available in most high-quality vitamins stores or on the Internet, in 500 mg capsules. We recommend taking two capsules per day with breakfast (one gram daily).

It is well known that the herb *gingko biloba* has a salutary effect on one's ability to concentrate and focus. Even the most recalcitrant skeptics have now conceded that the research does show improvement in mental function from this common and benign herbal medicine. One caveat, however, is for those cardiac patients who are on blood thinners, as gingko enhances the anticoagulant effect. That should be taken into account whenever there is testing or procedures to be performed. Simply mention to your doctor that you are taking it. A good dose is 160 mg of a 24 percent standardized leaf extract.

As a long-term herbal support, the sex gland driven endo-type often derives substantial benefit from the tonifier *ginseng*. There are many types of ginseng, but the most useful for this is the common Asian variety. Asian ginseng has an energizing quality for brain clarity, and it can be used in small amounts on a long-term basis.

Women might do a little better with the distaff sister of ginseng called dong quai, sometimes spelled tang kuei. It is an extremely useful addition to your program. As an adaptogen or tonifying agent at the same dose as ginseng above, this substance helps to balance a variety of metabolic processes. It is one of the most popular herbal items for women in all of Asia. (As with all herbs, consult a knowledgeable practitioner prior to taking when pregnant.)

Once again, let us remind you that vitamins, minerals, and amino acids are to be taken with food. Other products such as herbs and glandulars are more like medicines and should generally be taken on an empty stomach.

Exercise for the **Mental** Endo-Type

Your aerobic activity would best involve full awareness of where your body is and what it is doing. You are not really the best person to simply jog, amble, walk, or bike ride. A better activity for you would be dancing, martial arts, pilates, or yoga where there are formal steps involved, requiring your brain to be engaged, in order to follow.

The routines need not be cumbersome or complex, but they should allow you enough focus to keep your mind engaged on what is supposed to happen next. In this way you receive benefits of the exercise while also increasing your mental focus by connecting that exercise with an active mind.

You could perform some of the currently popular exercise forms of tai chi or chi gung. These involve a gradually learned series of very particular deliberate movements that require continued focus and concentration. The exercise they provide is beneficial, but even more so is that concentration of mental energy and focus that they involve.

The same holds true for slow stretching. Moving the joints slowly through their range of motion is indeed one of the healthiest activities you can do over the long haul, and is a perfect complement to the more rapid energy expenditure of aerobic exercise.

We've already extolled the virtues of yoga for the **mental** endo-type. There is yet another type of stretching recommended specifically for you, called gnana yoga, which means, "yoga of the mind." This is particularly helpful for the foggy sex-gland–driven endo-types, because it puts a spotlight on the actual thought processes that most of us take for granted. This is a true stretching, refocusing, and readjusting of the mind itself.

WHAT TO ADD

Mental Techniques

There are many ways to gain mastery over your mind. Remember that your mind is like a computer; you can be the one to program and operate it. Unruly minds make hasty decisions that may not have been carefully thought out. Your job is to learn to be the master of your mind.

Many people find it extremely helpful to reestablish regularly a connection with their surroundings, called grounding. A good exercise can be to sit comfortably, close your eyes, and take several deep cleansing breaths. Feel your feet planted firmly on the floor, and breathe deeply and fully.

As you breathe in, imagine that you have an opening in the center of the bottom of each foot. Breathing in, picture that you are drawing energy from the center of the Earth up through your feet. Some people find it helpful to imagine a cord, perhaps like a plant root, coming from the Earth and feeding energy into you. As you breathe in, draw Earth energy up through your feet, into your ankles, knees, thighs, hips, belly, chest, arms, neck, head, until you feel firmly planted and connected to the Earth. This kind of grounding exercise helps many scattered, fuzzy thinkers to clear their heads and feel connected and focused.

You might follow this with affirmations, such as "I feel centered and focused. My mind is clear, my thoughts are powerful," or "I am decisive and organized, and know from minute to minute exactly what needs to occur and when." Start saying, "I will remember things"; "I remember things clearly"; "I am sharp as a tack"; "I can easily remember peoples' names." These little visualization and affirmation tricks can help to improve your memory and focus enormously.

In addition to the memory and self-talk, realize that you are a fine person in the world, regardless of how your memory and thinking are performing currently. Try giving yourself appreciations, not just affirmations, but actual appreciation. This may include spending time each day reflecting on what you *have* accomplished, rather than focusing on what isn't going well. Considering everything you've been through, you are doing a good job just being here and trying your best.

Stress Reduction

Any yoga, stretching, or exercise can in general help you to reduce or manage stress. Certain highly effective activities, however, have the distinction of being called stress reduction modalities.

For **mental** endo-types, the best kind of stress reduction activity is a focused visual meditation. Simply sit comfortably, with eyes closed, and create the mental image of what you would like to see happen in your life. Be as specific and pointed as you possibly can. Be as hopeful and positive as you have ever been. See yourself more successful at work; see the details as to how that will unfold. See the office memos or newsletters touting your accomplishments. See your friends and loved ones congratulating you on how well you've been doing lately.

When this kind of activity is applied to an upcoming event, such as a job interview or company presentation, experts call it positive rehearsal, found to be very helpful for the person engaging in this activity. If you bring visual meditation into your life, it reminds and allows your brain to become a bit more focused, a little sharper.

If such visual images seem a little beyond you at this point, then start with a simple breathing exercise. Once again, sit comfortably with eyes closed. Feel the air in your chest as it moves in and out. Imagine the ribs and diaphragm expanding back and forth. See the blood mixing with the oxygen. Count how many seconds it takes for a slow deep breath to go fully in, and count how many seconds you can comfortably hold your breath before exhaling slowly back out. Count how many seconds it takes for a full exhale. Count the seconds you can wait before needing to inhale slowly once again.

Continue in this way for several minutes, and notice whether the number of counts for each of these separate aspects of breathing tends to change. In what way to do they change? Are you breathing deeper and slower, taking more counts? If so, how long does it take to really deepen your breathing? Can you feel the breath in the back of your throat as the air comes in through your nose? Can you feel your teeth as breath is exhaled through your mouth? And, all the while, keep asking yourself, "Why in the world am I doing this?"

Now, remind yourself that the reason you are doing this is to sharpen your ability to focus and concentrate on every aspect of your life, by practicing this focus on your breathing. Just as in the previous meditation where you imagined your life getting better, here the practice you get from being more focused will be of benefit to you in every facet of your life. These behaviors are a perfect antidote to foggy thinking!

Bodywork

A great type of bodywork for a **mental** endo-type is the discipline known as Feldenkrais. This is an example of participatory bodywork, rather than one in which the recipient is prone, passive, and quiet.

Here is an example of a Feldenkrais activity used in the practitioner's studio or for the recipient to do at home on his own. Arrange things so that you can lie facedown comfortably on a soft surface. Imagine a one-inch ball perched in the center of your back between your shoulder blades. Now, your task is to figure out which muscles to move, and how, to get that ball to move from the center of your spine over to your left shoulder without falling off.

The concentration required to figure out which muscle to move, and how much or little, and when to stop movement and start moving something else, engages the brain in a type of focus that then becomes generalized beyond the motor cortex. This type of training provides benefits to parts of the central nervous system that are not involved with muscle movement activity, but instead which are involved in keeping you clear-headed and on track.

Thus, here is a good maneuver for **mental** endo-types while getting any kind of massage or bodywork. Close your eyes and focus on exactly what it looks and feels like in that part of your body currently receiving treatment. This is the antidote to fuzzy, scattered, unfocused thinking. Like a lens that focuses light energy down to a point, which can then burn a hole through a piece of paper, you now have a lens that focuses your mental energy down to a point, keeping you from forgetting something important.

Other Enhancements

People who are in the **mental** endo-type category often derive great benefit from memory training, crossword puzzles, and trivia games. There is even a game called Concentration, where you pick up one of a number of facedown cards, turn it over, and try to recall where its match was located. Games such as these and other board or card games can be used to keep the mind engaged.

Aromatherapy

The most focusing and engaging scent to be utilized on a regular basis for the *high-testosterone* **mental** endo-type is rose. All over the world, this fragrance has been used to help bring a sometimes-scattered sex-hormone energy into a more clear focus. A small vial of rose scent can be carried around and sniffed several times a day to keep your brain awake and on track. (Never use aromatherapy oils in the mouth or on the tongue.)

- For *low testosterone*, an excellent aroma is sandlewood.
- For *high estrogen*, your aroma of choice might be cypress.
- For *low estrogen*, to boost mental clarity, try sage, which is considered to be particularly invigorating and helpful for focus.

Color Therapy

The long-term color choice for you, to bring greater focus and concentration, is orange. When you wake up and are still half-asleep, even the color of the orange juice helps bring you right back into alertness. Orange gets your attention; it's the color of pumpkins, warmth, heat, and sunrise. It is the color of the second chakra, down near where the sex glands are located.

Bach Flower Remedies

There are also specific flower remedies to help your **mental** endo-type maintain long-term focus and ability to concentrate. For high estrogen, try *holly* (four drops under tongue three times daily for a week). For low estrogen, try *wild oat* (same dosage). For high testosterone we suggest *vervain*, and for low testosterone try *mustard*.

Once again, the flower remedies are used once or twice a day when special focus is needed. They are taken by putting a few drops directly under the tongue or into a glass of drinking water. (Remember, flower remedies are used by mouth, but aromatherapy oils are only sniffed via the nose.)

Journaling

There is an old saying: "Those who forget are doomed to repeat." Keeping a journal can be extremely helpful, particularly if you pull out the old ones and periodically refresh yourself on past experiences and thoughts.

Diaries, poetry, and stories can be a healthy pastime for **mental** endo-types. Reflecting upon the present with the past in mind can be revelatory, and can save you from repeating mistakes.

Periodic evaluation of goals is also extremely useful, to remind you of what your intentions have been, and to redirect you during times of stress, when the mind may not be as clear as it should be.

In general, when you are under unusual stress, you may in fact find yourself feeling increasingly "fuzzy." It is precisely at these times that you would be well advised to use the tools suggested above.

Structured Environment

Sex hormone endo-types often have wonderful energy and creativity. Nevertheless, they often do their best work in a structured environment that helps keep their mind on track.

When considering your life path, or your next move, realize that a self-directed activity, like open-ended sales with a scattered client list, and payment only on commission may not be your best situation. It's not that all **mental** endo-types should necessarily punch a time clock, but having some orderly, easily understood expectations to fulfill generally works best for the long haul.

Those who are highly distractible may need to create for themselves situations that allow better focus. This can mean having one's own office, with a door, rather than a cubicle or open environment. They may have to let their supervisors know what they need or what will work best for them to ensure greater success. This might also include brief daily meetings with one's coworker or boss, in order to review the daily goals in a methodical manner. For foggy thinkers, a reliable environment that doesn't change much can help you stay focused and on target.

WHAT TO AVOID

In addition to some very general activities to avoid as listed below, the most specific concrete recommendation we would have for the foggy-thinking types would be to try to avoid unnecessary chemical exposures. Especially reduce your intake of mercury, almost ubiquitous in our environment at present, and a major cause of foggy thinking. The fish with the largest mercury content is swordfish, followed closely by halibut.

Tuna, a very popular staple in most households, has recently been found to contain worrisome high levels of mercury, to the extent that pregnant and childbearing age women are being advised to avoid it altogether. Sadly, we must concur that it would be wise for you to rotate the types of fish you eat, perhaps having only one serving per week of tuna (none for childbearing women).

We recommend avoiding contamination whenever possible, carefully considering your work and home locations in relation to Superfund sites, toxic dump sites, and pollution-spewing factories. Evaluate your living environment carefully to be sure you're not being unnecessarily exposed to airborne chemicals that can make you foggier, such as those emanating from glue on new carpeting, off-gassing of formaldehyde from new pressed-wood furniture, and freshly painted rooms.

Absolutely avoid exposure to insecticides or other forms of environmental estrogens, which just complicate your situation. Don't allow your home to be sprayed for ants or roaches. Instead, use pellets of boric acid mixed with peanut butter hidden behind furniture and on shelving. Use ant stakes or bait traps rather than having harmful sprays applied.

This brings up the topic of "smart nutrients" and "smart drugs." A whole industry has sprung up dealing with the "fogginess" that Americans are currently facing. Many of the items are extremely expensive and surrounded by hype that is neither accurate nor helpful.

Some of these may be worth a try if your hormones are balanced and you still need something extra to enhance mental performance. Remember, however, that strong nutraceuticals, and especially chemical medicines, used to alter brain function are not recommended for use on your own. We suggest that you avoid them entirely unless you have tried everything else mentioned previously, and now have the help of a careful and knowledgeable practitioner.

Avoid Disharmony and Scattered Energy

The last thing a **mental** endo-type person needs is to take a group of Cub Scouts to a park with no planned, structured activity for the day. The same would be true for taking your family on a trip to the circus, or to Disneyland. It's fine to do these things, but you might survive better with a conscious narrowing of the focus to one certain structured activity, like teaching the scouts how to build a campfire (safely, of course!).

At the circus, consider focusing only on what is going to happen in the main ring, or by spending time just in the Tomorrowland corner of Disneyland, rather than bouncing all around the park.

In fact, you may find it most helpful to your brain and hormones to focus on one project at a time. Carry it through to whatever state of completion you feel satisfied with, clean it up, and get out of that activity, and only then move on to the next activity. You will accomplish more, and do it better, with this kind of limited focus and discipline, which deeply suits your inner chemicals.

The same holds true for the number of activities that you put into any one day. Signing up for too many things to do is a common error for your endo-type, often leading to failure or distress. If you overburden yourself with high expectations and excess commitment, you will feel worse than if you set your goals simply and go about achieving them with grace and precision. This may mean saying no to extra requests made on your time; it can be difficult and disappointing, but in the long run, you will feel better about yourself and about what you have managed to accomplish.

Here's a final example. Some people watch television by channel surfing. They sit with the remote control and click through whatever happens to be on in their particular area of service. When something strikes their fancy, they watch for as long as it holds their interest, then click to the next channel. This is a kind of activity that **mental** endo-types should avoid! Your brain is already prone to getting distracted by one tangent or another; why train it to do this further? Instead (if you must watch television), pick up the television schedule before even turning on the set. If you find something that appeals strongly, make a point to tune in to it at the time it comes on, and then be sure to turn the television off right afterward.

In this way, you can practice keeping your mind on the task and on target. This is what will help you remember to pick your son up at the ballpark!

A ROAD MAP TO ENJOYING THE SEX GLAND–FRIENDLY LIFESTYLE

What works for the **mental** endo-type?

Many find it balancing and reassuring to surround themselves with beauty and order. Ambience is important to many people like yourself; adding beauty can be quite comforting, in the form of flowers, decoration, and furniture, arranging it to suit you. Clean off your desktop regularly. Straighten out your closet, and if you drive a lot, your car. This imposition of order helps your mind to declutter.

Mental endo-types often derive great pleasure from the use of music, aromas, colors, and other enhancements to empower their creative and sexual life. They can enjoy their sensuality, touching, tasting, feeling things around them, to help restore that hormonal balance.

Remember, lastly, that balance is the key to unleashing the creative and powerful life force from within you. Using this knowledge wisely can allow you to have years of sexual fulfillment, as well as the joy of being a productive, contributing, accomplishing person in the world.

CONCEPT SUMMARY

1. Schedule short meditative times into your life. Visualization, imagery, and other mind techniques can help you stay focused.
2. The body chemistry is known to be very responsive to emotions and their resultant thought patterns. Affirmations, self-appreciation, and grounding are excellent tools to support mental clarity.

ACTION SUMMARY

❑ Gradually shift your exercise efforts toward focused stretching like yoga or tai chi and aerobics like dance or martial arts.

❑ Use imagery, self-appreciation, and visualization to improve mental clarity. Include breathing exercises and mantra meditation to sharpen concentration.

❑ Seek out gentle structured bodywork like Feldenkrais, using the mind to focus on the body part receiving attention.

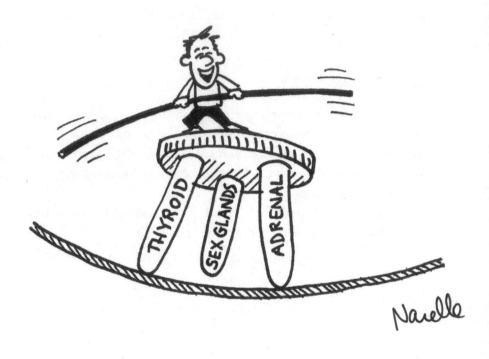

CHAPTER 11

STAY CALM AND CENTERED WHILE ENJOYING LIFE
RELAXATION TECHNIQUES FOR HORMONAL HARMONY

There is no joy, but calm!

—Alfred, Lord Tennyson

Although the frazzled and stressed-out Emily had begun to feel much more like her old self, she also knew enough about health to realize that such benefits are all too often short-lived. Emily was a practical and diligent person. She was cautious in her stock brokerage advice, and very sensible with her own small portfolio. She was a no-nonsense girl who now came to the clinic wanting to know how she could maintain her sense of well being for the long term.

Discussing the categories of nutrition, exercise, and stress reduction, we suggested her next step was to veer away from junk foods and into calmer kinds of intake. Always on the go, she had generally settled for prepackaged foods and quick meals except for those occasions when she met with clients for lunch. Sometimes her days were so busy that she settled for a fast microwave dish at the office, while continuing her work.

We explained to her that this way of eating resulted in increased tension and stress, suggesting instead that she invest a little more time into preparing higher-quality foods. The fresh grains and vegetables we recommended would have fewer chemicals than packaged items, also providing a much more even-running metabolism.

The final long-term recommendation came for Emily only at a much later time. Based on her self-evaluations and testing, we were able to suggest to Emily that her main stressor was the underlying sense of urgency she lived with continuously, combined with the need she felt to be perfect. The intervention for these deeply rooted personality traits would first involve an openness to books and practitioners, in order to develop a positive change in attitude. She began to understand that it was okay to strive, to be always on time, and to be as good as she could be, without having to be so uptight about the outcome. It was okay to push, but she could become more relaxed about how things would eventually work out, knowing that in the end, she did not have total control over them.

Her mantra became "You win some, and lose some;" this little phrase, oddly enough, gave her more comfort and peace, in the same exact work and family setting. Emily's change of heart made a major difference, eventually directing her body chemicals into something more useful and less distressing.

LONG-TERM CHALLENGES OF THE EMOTIONAL ENDO-TYPE

As we've said, adrenal-driven types are often angry, irritable, worried, or fearful. They have a tendency toward phobias and panic disorders. Often when they come to doctors' offices seeking help, they are diagnosed with anxiety or depression, and treated with psychotropic drugs. Their situation is not thought of as an endocrine challenge, but rather as a psychological problem. When on occasion an endocrine problem is considered, the treatment is generally as follows: "You're low in estrogen; here's a prescription."

With the premature cessation of the Women's Health Initiative study due to the serious deleterious side effects of estrogen, women were left with a void in treatment for these physical/mental/emotional concerns. Our best solution is to encourage you look carefully at your endocrine glands, especially thyroid, adrenal, and sex hormone–producing glands, and to determine which require rebalancing, and especially in what order. For those experiencing anger, agitation, anxiety, or similar behaviors, we find that adrenal balancing can often be surprisingly helpful.

> If you are an adrenal-driven endo-type, your long-
> term health and balance will depend upon being
> sure that your adrenaline and cortisol levels stay
> within a comfortable range and balance.

As mentioned in chapter 7, adrenaline increases jittery feelings, nervousness, anxiety, worry, and rage. At its worst, it can result in paranoia. People with high levels of adrenaline can come across as bullies, when what is more accurate is that they are driving themselves too hard, thereby becoming irritable.

OPTIMAL APPROACHES FOR LONG-TERM SUCCESS

How can you avoid these unsatisfying behavior patterns? Once you have dealt with the immediate situation, you will need to overcome some longer-term natural inclinations by modifying your habits.

Improving Your Relationship with Stress

This simple-sounding advice may be the hardest thing for you to do, if you—like millions of other **emotional** endo-types—are hooked on adrenaline. We have learned to push these little glands to get us further, allowing ambition to overshadow simple common sense. It is critical for the adrenal-challenged to find enjoyable activities and to slow down! Make time for things you love, including people, pets, nature, and hobbies.

Unconscious ambition is generally what drives us to take on more than we can handle. Many times just shining the light of reason on these ingrained, repetitious habits can help them to lose force, and to be replaced by a healthier decision-making process.

Therefore, here's the very first approach that you will find useful for the long-term, now that your glands are somewhat rebalanced:

> Decrease the sources of stress in your life, so that you don't
> keep knocking your system out of balance over and over.

This requires some careful thought, because the sources and origin of stress are different for everyone. What we are really talking about here is learning more specifically what sorts of people, activities, intake, or output causes you distress, and making adjustments accordingly.

Some of these can be changed, but some can't. The French have a saying: "What cannot be cured must be endured." For things that cannot be easily changed, we here suggest that you devise your best tactics for enduring these stressors more gracefully. Your goal, of course, is to reduce their impact on you while learning to deal with them more appropriately. In other words, you also need to develop new approaches for dealing with the *effects* of stress on your system.

Strategic Planning

If you know that you are an adrenal-driven endo-type, regardless of how well you may be balanced from specific maneuvers presented in chapter 7, there is a certain amount of strategic planning you will find very useful for the long haul.

You must first realize something very important about yourself:

You have to intervene earlier, and cannot allow things to build up.

You are dealing with chemicals that—when you face unexpected stress—can quickly upset your balance.

What does this look like? It means that as soon as you feel your muscles getting a little tighter, as soon as you sense your mind starting to race, as soon as there's the least bit of that frazzled feeling, you *immediately* stop and take stock of yourself.

You then say, "Aha, this is exactly what I am supposed to look out for. Now that I see it, I'm going to take a few slow breaths, and decide that I'm going to turn this around. Then I am going to ask myself, what else is needed? What do I need to do? I'm starting to get fearful, or angry—what will help this situation?"

This maneuver is called preemptory management, intended to prevent the cascade that will eventually spin out of control. It is the way to minimize a chemical secretion that starts as a small snowball and ends up an avalanche.

Whenever possible, you must attempt to manage or avoid anything that increases the potential for escalation. Notice your early warning signals, and interrupt the cycle of escalation. In other words, preemptory avoidance is healthy here! It is a way for you to manage your own stress by taking charge of situations to the best of your ability.

WHAT TO CONTINUE

Nutrition

You will likely find it useful to continue your dietary focus on a slow-burning, balanced, and middle-of-the-road approach to protein and complex carbohydrates. You have seen how strongly the **emotional** endo-type is prone to hypoglycemia. If you want to achieve a long-term improvement in your life balance, you have to grab the "cookie monster" by the ears and wrestle him to the ground. In other words, gradually reduce then eliminate completely refined carbs and sugar.

You may need help making dietary changes, and plenty of guidance is available in the form of nutritional advisors, individual counseling, and groups. Some of our patients did not get a handle on their sweet tooth issues until joining Overeaters Anonymous or Food Addicts Anonymous. Others find relief using totally regimented diet plans, such as Jenny Craig or Weight Watchers, which can reeducate you on your relationship with food.

Adrenal types need much more vitamin C than can normally be obtained from foods; for this reason we recommend continuing vitamin C in the amounts discussed in chapter 8.

In general, adrenal-driven endo-types need to eat more frequently than other people. The standard three-meals-a-day routine doesn't suit you as well as smaller, more frequent meals. We suggest a light breakfast like unsweetened oatmeal, including a breakfast protein, such as lean meat, fish patty, or whey protein shake.

Then comes a midmorning snack, around 10:30 or so. This can involve eating some nuts or whole grain crackers or both. You can put a simple nut butter on the crackers for additional protein value.

Lunch can occur at a regular time, possibly salad and fish, as a prelude to a midafternoon snack, around 2:30 or 3 p.m. Again, this snack can involve crackers and nuts or nut butter. Some folks do well with a low-fat cheese or unsweetened yogurt at this time.

For dinner, again we advise smaller portions than standard American fare, at the usual time. If you notice hunger by bedtime, a small snack can be helpful to keep your body nourished until morning. These five or six small meals a day can help you to feel more leveled out, steadier over the long haul.

Supplemental Nutrients

As far as *vitamins* are concerned, the major item you should continue to take in high levels on an ongoing basis is the B vitamin pantothenic acid. Be sure to include 500 mg every morning. This vitamin is intimately involved with the energy balance of normal adrenal function.

For the adrenal type, the most important *mineral* for your type of challenge is higher than usually suggested levels of chromium. This is the mineral intimately involved in carbohydrate metabolism, similar to iron's involvement to oxygen respiration, and the one you could add for the long haul, at a dose of about 200 to 300 mcg per day on an ongoing basis.

The most important amino acid to add is *tyrosine*. This generally comes as one capsule of 500 mg, and we recommend that you take this daily with your multivitamin and chromium. Remember that tyrosine is the basic skeletal structure, or precursor for several adrenal hormones.

Exercise

The best body movement for the **emotional** endo-type is just the right amount of comfortable enjoyable *aerobic activity*. It could be anything from a five-minute brisk walk every other day to a fifty-minute strenuous workout every single day. Seek out and find what pleases your adrenal system most.

Adrenal types tend to do quite well with vigorous or competitive exercise to burn off some of the hard-to-eliminate buildup of excess adrenal hormones. Keep in mind that if you are in adrenal excess, you're running a lot of adrenaline. This can make you very jittery.

Tennis or basketball can be very helpful. Stretching can be more active, and for those who enjoy it, try to add more vigorous martial arts. These can include tai chi, or the newly popularized shaolin, aikido, karate, or boxing. Some even like using a punching bag or chopping wood, all of which will burn up excess energy.

There is one exception to this rule: Not everyone who is an adrenal endo-type needs vigorous activity to burn off excess hormone. In fact, if you are completely adrenal exhausted (Stage III adrenal failure), you need to conserve your energy.

In this situation, vigorous exercise can actually make you feel worse, by draining you when you are already depleted. Exceeding these suggested amounts of exercise if you are an **emotional** endo-type is often maladaptive. This means it can result in diminishing returns and even make things worse. Following these guidelines, on the other hand, can lead to a comfortable sense of release and balance.

The solution here is to do something that will invigorate your system without exhausting it. Eventually, as the adrenals improve, the amount of exercise can be increased both in duration and intensity.

WHAT TO ADD

For those eager to embark on the long-term adrenal-sustaining maneuvers, we can suggest that you consider using some of the following gentle approaches.

Just as crucial as exercise guidelines are the specific tools of effective stress reduction. We have mentioned the benefits of paying attention to causes and effects of stress, and why it is absolutely essential for **emotional** endo-types to manage stress more gracefully.

Specific Ways to Minimize the Causes of Your Stress

If there are particular activities or people in your life that you know are perceived as very stressful by your system, it would behoove you to minimize your exposure to them, at least for the duration of the initial rebalancing that we are recommending in this chapter.

We realize that in "real life," this is not always possible, but you need to do your best. If it is an interpersonal problem, try discussing it with the other person in terms of your health needs. Also, you can remove yourself from the situation by being around less, whenever possible. Set firm clear boundaries to reduce your stress.

Specific Ways to Minimize the Effects of Stress

Next, you can adapt to the situation by altering your own internal mechanisms to reduce your biochemical fallout. Sometimes, this might mean putting in earplugs, whether actual or metaphorical.

Commonly, people make the mistake of using a tranquilizer that can further upset metabolic balance, and can also be addictive. Far better would be to utilize milder yet effective relaxing herbs, such as valerian root, hops, passion flower, or lady slipper. These can be found individually or in combination at good health food stores.

One frequently successful maneuver for stress reduction is meditation. This activity reduces both the causes, and the effects, of stress. It can be performed during small increments of time throughout the day, and does not necessarily require any special equipment or training. We recommend it as part of every stress-reduction program.

As we suggested for Emily, it can be good to do a walking meditation. The reason for this is that often an adrenal endo-type is a person who could benefit from meditation but has a hard time sitting still. This person does better when moving. It seems to go against his or her grain just to sit and do nothing, which can sometimes be perceived as additional stress.

This walking meditation also engages the brain. (The adrenal endo-types don't like to clear their mind and be free of all thought—it's either irritating or frightening to them.) A type of meditation that involves moving the body helps the thoughts to move gently, too, perhaps allowing greater processing, particularly when breathing deeply as you walk.

Sometimes the effect of the stress is to tighten the muscles. The purpose of adrenaline is to increase blood flow to certain areas, so that the muscles can be activated for fight or flight. If, however, you are not fighting or fleeing, but instead just have too much stress from your work, you can end up with heightened activity in your muscles. This can result in your becoming tight, sore, and uncomfortable. Walking, deep breathing, and relaxation will help.

Stretching

What type of stretching activities might be best in the long run for an adrenal driven type? These are generally more active than the typical yoga postures. An adrenal person might do well with fast stretching, where the limbs are put through their range of motion in fairly deliberate and rapid ways. It is often very appealing to the antsy adrenal type. Again a specific example is the shaolin martial arts form, often described as very rapid and vigorous tai chi.

Bodywork

Many different types of bodywork are appropriate for the adrenal-driven person. Some of the most effective, however, would be those that are more deep-tissue than Swedish massage. Deep-tissue massage usually requires a specially trained practitioner who is skilled in a school of this kind of deep-tissue, emotional-release bodywork, such as Rolfing, Hellerwork, Trager work, Aston-Patterning, LooyenWork, and others, mostly originating on the West Coast of the United States or in Europe. The maneuvering can look like massage at first glance, or physical therapy, because the practitioner stands and the recipient is flat on a table. The actual activity, however, is quite different from either massage or physical therapy. Parts of the practitioner's body, such as fingertips, knuckles, and elbows are applied with enough force to the recipient to evoke a different type of response than the usual massage strokes. It can at times be uncomfortable enough to border on pain, as very tight musculature and connective tissue is pressed upon, mobilized, and loosened.

In addition to loosening some of the internal structures, a common result of this activity is the evoking of certain feelings and memories, accompanied by vocalization of sounds. The actual sounds can be anything from *ahhh* or *owww* to full sentences of stored emotion, sometimes even accompanied by a flood of either tears or laughter. This aspect is called emotional release, and although a useful therapeutic maneuver for any brave soul, it is especially helpful for adrenal-driven types.

Additional Creative Tools

Aromatherapy

The **emotional** endo-type does well with *lavender*, which is somewhat calming to most people. Adrenal types find it particularly relaxing and centering, perhaps because it activates a center of the brain over which they have less control. While most people might use a sniff of lavender under their nose to fall asleep more easily, an adrenal type does well to carry lavender around with her, taking periodic whiffs throughout the day.

Colors

The color most helpful for dealing with adrenal issues is yellow, the color of canaries, lemons, a candle flame, and the noonday sun. Yellow is warm and restful, and can signify that all is well. Yellow is also the color of the traffic light that says proceed with caution, neither completely stop nor freely go, neither fight nor flight mode.

Flower Remedies

This treatment is very restorative and balancing. The remedies are extracts made of specific flowers known to have certain qualities that match your need. Most famous is Bach's *Rescue Remedy*, a combination of various flower extracts used as an emergency pick-me-up. A person who has just received bad news often finds that Rescue Remedy, either dropped under the tongue or put into drinking water, helps to restore a sense of peace and ease during stress.

Also recommended is *olive* for those feeling depleted from a long period of giving to others, *oak* for those who notice despondency and a feeling that they can't go on. These are very helpful to sensitive **emotional** endo-types, and can be used regularly to help the person enjoy a more complete range of emotional balance and of calm times, as well.

Special Counseling

In addition to the nutrition, exercise, stress reduction, and bodywork, there is another area of activity that can be helpful for both the causes and the effects of stress. Being a less worried, less tense person involves exploration of the psychological and spiritual aspects of life. Adrenal abnormalities are sometimes the result of external factors, such as pollution and economic downturn. Often, however, they are due to internal factors, more related to family of origin issues, causing deep-seated anger and disappointment.

If this is part of your situation, you might need to learn techniques for safe emotional discharge, rather than let these feelings continue to affect your health. Most of us need help in working on these issues with good books, good programs, and good practitioners. All this can be an important part of your stress reduction program.

Not every counselor is right for each person; for this reason, there are many types of counseling, and therapy, some very active, some passive, some noisy, some meditative.

In general, **emotional** endo-types may need to start with a therapist who can initally keep pace with their rapid emotional timing, and then gradually move them to a more peaceful and harmonious state.

This pacing maneuver is prominent in neurolinguistic programming, a type of therapy wherein the therapist mirrors the client, and as trust develops, is able to move the pacing to something more relaxing and healing. Some therapies are physically active, involving moving around the room, expressing through postures and body movements, making sounds, encouraging emotion. Some are more mental, which would be best suited for the sex-hormone types who need more mental focus. Some can be deeply relaxing, others energizing. A good counselor or therapist learns to set the tone for pacing according to the needs of the person in front of him or her.

Some sessions can involve role-playing, bringing the person back to an earlier time in her life, or to a future event that may provoke anxiety and allow for positive rehearsal. There are countless types of therapy, so we encourage you to become acquainted with these systems and find out which attract you, which repel you, and perhaps even which bore you. Your feelings may indicate directions for work to be accomplished, and in the hands of a well-trained therapist, the pacing will match your needs.

Many people find great benefit in short-term therapy interventions, going for a brief time during crises to find emotional balance. Others feel they have long stored emotional baggage, some quite traumatic, and realize they will need to be involved for the longer term in counseling endeavors. Many find they can touch in and out as they feel the need, relying on their own internal drive to decide when they require a tune-up.

Finally, our time-saving devices (ha!) have lured us into a false complacency, inspiring us to believe that we will get more done in less time, when what actually occurs instead is that we commit to more than could possibly be done. Adrenal types need to be especially on guard against overly committing.

Surround yourself with loved ones and upbeat people. Take regular quiet time for deep breathing, relaxation exercises, stretching, and connecting to nature. Journaling can help to relieve inner feelings, writing only for yourself. Your connection to your creativity can unleash a vast potential, as long as you direct this energy properly.

Altruistic behaviors, such as providing help and healing to others, can actually be very restorative to the self as long as you have taken care of yourself first. Focus on what you want to become.

Ultimately, these types of support can result in putting you back in the driver's seat, in charge of your life, and being successful.

WHAT TO AVOID

The **emotional** endo-types, nutritionally speaking, do best to avoid extra stimulation.

Foods

This generally means toning down the spice on your foods, not eating very hot or very cold foods and avoiding too much sugar. This does not mean eating only very bland foods. As mentioned previously, an adrenal-driven **emotional** endo-type may need more salt than the average person. Keeping a salt shaker on the table is a fine idea, so long as your blood pressure stays normal.

The reason for this is that when the adrenal is in its most common abnormal state of insufficiency, it is common to have an altered amount of the adrenal hormone aldosterone, resulting in an extra large release of salt by the kidney, causing relative salt depletion and lowered blood pressure.

Certain People

Regarding relationships, we recommend that this endo type do everything possible to avoid vexing, angry people. We realize that each of us can sometimes come across like this, but there are some people who have a constant chip on their shoulder, who are ready to lose control with only slight provocation. To the extent that it is possible, try to steer clear of these people, who can easily aggravate your own hair-trigger tendencies.

Remember that being an **emotional** endo-type means that sometimes it takes very little to elicit a massive, inappropriate response. Knowing this about your present state, it is wise to surround yourself with more calm, serene people.

Action Movies and Too Much TV News

Today's top thrillers carry an extreme amount of adrenaline punch. The sophistication of camera techniques and special effects are quite sufficient to raise and lower your adrenaline and cortisol levels drastically, in alternating fashion for the entire duration of the movie.

The exquisitely delicate interacting molecules of your hormone system were not really made for this constant barrage of high-level stimulation.

While some people find action movies fun and have gotten into the habit of using thrillers to feel more alive, adrenal-challenged people could do themselves a favor by trying this experiment. Spend a week without watching thriller movies or television, or listening to loud jumpy music driven by heavy bass. Attend gatherings that include only a few people at a time (as opposed to seventy thousand at a football game, or even seventy at a noisy bar). Avoid the flashing-light discotheque, and refrain from ingesting the usual stimulants.

See if after that week your nervous system and your emotions are more even and comfortable. You may actually notice feeling very tired. This is not boredom, but instead a signal that you have been overamping and overrevving your particular system, and that you need some rest to recharge.

Psychoactive Drugs

It is common for the adrenal-driven **emotional** endo-type to resort to either uppers or downers of some sort, maybe over-the-counter or sometimes prescription versions. This is because their energy has generally been on a roller coaster, hyped up, or crashing.

People who have a hard time getting up in the morning because of their adrenal status, or whose energy has crashed after an excessively strenuous episode of fight or flight, will often find the hit of caffeine, ma huang, or something stronger to be quite attractive. The problem is, the use of these products just perpetuates the cycle, keeping you locked into an unbalanced hormonal roller coaster.

Some folks, when too hyped up, will then use chemical downers, like valium or alcohol, to "wind down" after having spent a full day unnecessarily stressing themselves with spicy food, caffeine, hours of TV news, and a long action movie.

It is much better for your overall health to direct your life onto a more level track, rather than a roller coaster. You will live longer, better, happier, and more fulfilled.

Betting, Gambling, or Risk Taking

One of the worst activities for adrenal types is engaging in betting large amounts of your money on daily life events, like sports or races. We're not talking about the occasional lottery ticket, or playing cards with friends for small stakes.

What we are referring to is wagering any important amount of your money on whether Miami beats Denver. This raises your adrenaline levels unnecessarily, making the game a stressful event instead of an interesting pastime. It may be an activity that some are truly addicted to, but most people gamble because others are doing it and seem to enjoy it, and they think its fun. It's actually not so much fun for the adrenal-driven endo-type, when it is perceived internally as stressful. Ideally you would determine and wager only what is an insignificant amount of cash, the gain or loss of which would not be at all stressful for you.

A ROAD MAP TO THE ADRENAL-FRIENDLY LIFESTYLE

With these basic recommendations, the **emotional** endo-type person can look forward to a much more comfortable existence. You can go through life without having the white knuckles and clenched fists so common in previous years. You can enjoy other people more; they can enjoy you more. You will sleep better at night and wake up more easily in the morning.

Think about what it will be like to feel that you have enough time for things you want to do each day. Consider how much more comfortable it would be to enjoy what your coworkers do, rather than being annoyed by them. Think of how this could change your life.

Now you can look forward to the future, not with dread of all the things that could go wrong, but with eager anticipation of things going well. It can be the difference between often being afraid or annoyed versus generally being pleased with yourself and the world.

CONCEPT SUMMARY

1. If you are an **emotional** endo-type, your long-term balance will depend upon being sure that your adrenaline and cortisol levels stay within a comfortable range.
2. Decreasing the sources of stress in your life will help prevent knocking your system out of balance over and over.
3. Learning to intervene earlier helps keep stresses from building up.
4. When seeking counseling, remember that not every counselor is right for each person. There are many types of counseling and therapy, some more active, some more reflective.
5. Rather than being fearful or irritated, you can be calmer, happier, and more fun to be around.

ACTION SUMMARY

❑ Continue to eat a middle-of-the-road balance of protein and slowburning *complex carbohydrates*, and a to eat more *frequent, smaller meals*.

❑ Stay at high levels of B-vitamin pantothenic acid (500 mg daily), continue the mineral *chromium* (200 to 300 mcg daily), and take the amino acid *tyrosine* (500 mg daily).

❑ In place of tranquilizers, try using combinations of these herbs: valerian root, hops, passion flower, or lady slipper (two to three capsules taken two or three times daily).

❑ Stick with *vigorous, aerobic exercise* (except if your saliva test reveals stage III adrenal exhaustion, then do only *very brief* mild workouts).

❑ Add more active stretching to your regular program.

❑ Do some deep-tissue bodywork such as Rolfing, Hellerwork, or Aston Patterning (see "Finding Appropriate Practitioners" in Appendices on page 273), preferably a type that allows for emotional release.

❑ A "moving meditation" can be just the thing for the adrenal compromised person. Keep the mind and body active, and remember to breathe deeply and fully.

❑ *Add Complementary Therapies*
    ❑ Aromatherapy—Lavender (calming)
    ❑ Color therapy—Yellow (restful)
    ❑ Flower remedies
        ❑ olive for ongoing tiring challenges
        ❑ oak when you feel you can't go on

❑ *Avoid or Decrease*
    ❑ Extra stimulation
    ❑ Angry, vexing people
    ❑ Scary television/movies
    ❑ Stimulants and downers (tranquilizers)
    ❑ Betting, gambling, or risk taking

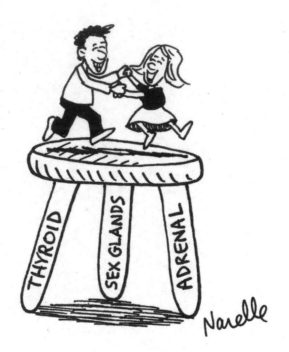

CHAPTER 12

PUTTING IT TOGETHER

Beside the lake, beneath the trees . . . and dancing in the breeze.

—William Wordsworth

Phoebe, Meredith, and Emily were relaxing together at a local restaurant. Meredith especially was a bit tired, having just assisted in teaching two yoga classes at the nearby center. The live music for the night was a guitar player who was just warming up. The way he was tuning his guitar caught their attention.

He was playing the same chord, over and over, while tuning individual strings. First he would pick each of the three strings of the chord individually. Then he played the whole chord of all three strings simultaneously. Next he would adjust one of the strings and repeat the process again, first each string individually, then all three combined. At every step of this process he listened intently.

Each well-tuned note evidently made a satisfactory sound, but richer, fuller and more vibrant was the beautiful sound made when all three strings of the chord were played together. For this musician, it was evidently here that the exquisite depths of harmonies and overtones truly emerged.

Our three ladies were riveted by this. Each, in her own timing, realized how balance and fine-tuning can create exquisite results.

By now it should be abundantly clear that these three women, and even you, are most likely a *mix* of these three endo-types, if not right at this moment, then possibly at a different stage of your life. Up until now, their stories have purposely been presented to portray an archetype of each endo-type, how the pure essence of that gland imbalance might present itself.

Life, however, is not as neatly packaged as this construct, and further gland balancing will require you to use some flexibility and intuition, for best results. The three major glands do not act singly, nor do they simply influence us individually.

Each one of us, and every symptom we experience, is actually a result of a unique divine mix. The three regulatory hormones each works in conjunction with the others. You cannot adjust any one of them without soon taking the others into account. Your goal is to find that place where your hormonal health strikes a rich and resonant chord.

RELATED HORMONAL INTERACTIONS

Remember that it is not just these three hormones that are at work in our bodies. As we've said at various times throughout this book, doing something good somewhere eventually helps everything everywhere. Taking in proper nutrients allows many of the other hormones to do their work more harmoniously. The same is true for good stress reduction and exercise. Having assessed your levels by self-evaluation questionnaires and saliva, you now have a road map for how to proceed, even if your endo-type changes over time. This chapter will provide the details.

In addition to our three main hormones, there is growth hormone, which regulates certain aspects of metabolic activity. The hormone insulin controls how much carbohydrate is available to enter our cells. An alteration of this process is the recently elucidated and surprisingly common syndrome X, wherein there is insulin resistance along with high blood pressure, central obesity, polycystic ovaries. Melatonin is intimately involved with our sleeping and waking cycles. The list includes perhaps twenty others, all of which can be major players at one time or another.

**Our point has been that this amazingly grand
complex of messenger molecules works
better when your three "energy" hormones
are balanced and in their proper ratios.**

In addition to causing the symptoms of feeling fat, fuzzy, or frazzled, our individual hormonal balance is also a major contributor to other illnesses that can affect us in various ways. Infertility, endometriosis, recurrent miscarriage, serious ovarian and breast cysts, even breast cancer can be related to your hormonal balance.

Nor is it just women who are affected by these hormonal imbalances. Heart disease, arthritis, and prostate problems likewise have a strong hormonal connection. Early in this new century, major European research known as the Rotterdam Study evaluated 10,994 men and women aged fifty-five plus over a ten-year period to investigate and observe the prevalence and incidence of risk factors for chronic diseases in the elderly. Its findings demonstrated that low thyroid is a separate independent risk factor for cardiac illness and stroke in elderly women. Recent studies have confirmed these findings for men as well. Moreover, younger age groups were similarly affected.

Depression, personality disorder, paranoia, and schizophrenia are serious psychiatric conditions that are known to have a hormonal cause rather than a purely psychiatric one. In fact, many more major illnesses than could be easily listed here are related to this vital balance.

CHANGE YOUR HORMONES, CHANGE THE WORLD

The mind is our greatest healing tool. It directs the activity for everything in the body, largely via our hormones. In order to make the kind of changes that are necessary to reclaim your health and to stay well, you will need to rearrange some thoughts and behaviors.

If you plan to first change your hormones and then the world, you will need to know more about the nature of true and lasting change. In fact, you need to embrace a closely related concept, that of *empowerment*. This means you start with healing yourself, then, when you feel much better, you can join with others to begin to make a difference in the world. Taken together, these two concepts can indeed change your life *and* change the world.

Empowerment and the Balance of Life

Empowerment is the art of living your life fully, claiming all your innate strength and skill to enhance your own well-being and that of the world we share. It is like a yoga practice, wherein one learns to test one's boundaries, stretch and be flexible, all the while strengthening your inner core.

"Power" has been defined in many ways: the ability to influence change, to have whatever it is you want, and to have influence. People may access their internal power using a variety of tools, including mental exercise, physical exercise, education, religion, and in general through being curious and in contact with many people, places, or things. Life itself can be a grand and rewarding journey when approached with openness and a willingness to grow and change. Empowerment occurs when you utilize all your strengths, skills, and knowledge to get the desired results.

These concepts can be applied to every arena of your life, but here we are especially referring to the process of healing your glands. As you empower yourself and heal your biochemistry, you will be in a much better position to do good work in the world. Start with *you* first!

How to Proceed for Multigland Involvement

Having addressed your major imbalance, you are now in a position to take the other glands into account. Determining your endo-type in chapters 3 and 4 has guided your rebalancing efforts as to which gland to tackle first. Now, that same data can guide your choice about which gland to tackle next.

Returning to full hormonal balance often requires attention to more than one gland. It is important to tackle them in the order in which they guide you. Learning to listen to your unique hormone chemistry, with its very specific calls, messages, and clues, can become a model for how you live your life. Following your instincts, combined with your practitioner's wisdom, is the best way to proceed.

If your self-evaluations and home lab tests did not show a runaway favorite in the form of a clear, single-gland issue, then you are especially liable to derive further benefit from the mixed approach. A great many people are mixed endo-types. They are, for example, mainly low thyroid but also high adrenal. This is a very common situation today given the endogenous (stress) and exogenous (pollution) causes as explained in chapter 2.

Other people might be mainly high sex-gland, but also low adrenal. In fact, there are twenty-seven different possible combinations, if you consider three different levels of severity (high, low, and normal) for three different glands (thyroid, adrenal, sex), and three possible orders of presentation (which presents as primary, which secondary, and which tertiary).

Your main influence determines whether you are a **physical, mental,** or **emotional** endo-type. These major imbalances are best handled first, and hopefully by now you have successfully done so.

Dealing with Secondary Imbalances

Should you decide that you now want or need to do some fine-tuning, merely go back to the appropriate chapters that cover your secondary issue. Here you will find plenty of rebalancing tools to add to your existing program. Once again we remind you to move cautiously, one step at a time, giving your body a chance to adjust to the new interventions. In most cases, adding a new supplement will not interfere with your existing program. If it does affect you adversely, stop whatever new supplement you are taking and move on to something else.

Primary rebalancing is like taking your car in for a safety check and oil change. Secondary rebalancing is more like having a full tune-up. What would tertiary rebalancing be like? This is when you pay close attention to all three glands, in the order suggested, through your self-evaluations and home tests. We like to call this full program a complete overhaul.

We Are All Canaries!

This book was especially written to capture the attention and imagination of those who could immediately relate to the title, feeling fat, fuzzy, or frazzled. The overarching reality, however, is that most humans are likely to be impacted by the growing numbers of hormone-mimicking substances flooding our living, breathing planet. It is possible that many of the people you know might also benefit from reading this book.

Most of us do not have all three major symptoms, but instead have multiple other symptoms that could well be related to energy hormone imbalances. Of particular relevance seem to be the preponderance of annoying skin conditions, mental or psychological disturbances, and other autoimmune conditions that are being made worse by tired glands. Related symptoms can range from cracking nails or hair falling out to a thick, frequently bitten tongue, from Reynaud's syndrome (which is when your fingers turn blue or white when exposed to cold) to worsened diabetes, low libido to high cholesterol.

Without proper diagnosis, we will never know how many people are plagued with an underlying, undermining hormonal excess or deficit condition. Many will be treated symptomatically, caught in a revolving door between various doctors' offices, clinics, and hospitals. It is certainly our hope they find their way to useful information and are given the chance to feel better again.

If this book reminds you of people you know, you might want to tell them about it, or even give them a copy. While these ideas are not always easy concepts to grasp, and can't be easily explained in a few words, they do make sense when put in the context of the larger picture, which we have attempted to share here.

We certainly believe that our overwhelmed medical system would be less burdened, and perhaps be more effective and responsive, if it weren't so bogged down by the millions who are out of balance and just feel lousy. Our combined sixty-plus years of experience (our hormone-balancing efforts keep us young!) suggests the following:

**This one previously undefined problem,
hormonal imbalance, when fixed, can ameliorate
hundreds of other conditions.**

This could then release doctors to provide better care for more clear syndromes and ailments. In other words, these hormonal difficulties might be undermining our collective health, causing frustration on the part of caregivers and consumers.

The canaries in the coal mines, you might recall, died from inhalation of unseen gas. We human canaries need to become more vigilant about our symptoms and their patterns. We need to find new ways to evaluate and command better care in a gasping health-care system that will not hear our concerns, but must be encouraged to listen nonetheless. In addition to paying attention, those who feel improved after hormone rebalancing need to become louder and more outspoken, sharing their knowledge in public arenas where health or environmental discussions are taking place.

How would you begin to share your information to the benefit of not only yourself and loved ones, but also to help our national and international communities? You need only use your personal experience as testimony, to find powerful arenas and methods for sharing the ideas you have discovered here.

To simplify that process, we are using this final chapter to empower you as a health advocate, whether you wish to advocate further for yourself only or for the entire planet, and for all those beautiful life-forms on it.

Sensitive People Need Sensitive Medicines

Starting with some basic review of what we have presented, keep in mind that those who are serving as canaries for this life-draining situation need *not* wait until they hover near death's door before offering a warning. If you have found relief from any of the ideas presented here, you might start trying to catch the attention of friends and family.

So, the next time a colleague tells you about her hair falling out, inexplicable weight gain, extreme agitation or irritability, or confides in you about low libido or repeated miscarriage, we hope you will advise her to get her glands checked very carefully.

Our program encourages health consumers to become aware sooner of possible gland sluggishness, in order to employ remedies before this condition has a chance to wreak further havoc on your body and your life. These remedial measures, when taken early, will be less drastic, less invasive, and more effective. Early intervention is a key to an easier success.

As Phoebe, Meredith, and Emily had started to feel well again, their family, friends, and coworkers noticed. Soon after, others approached them with their personal stories of feeling fat, fuzzy, and frazzled. They clearly hoped for validation that there actually was something wrong with them physically, that they were not simply crazy, and that there was something that could be done to help them. As the three women shared their stories with others, they began to sound like experts in their own right. This gave them pleasure, realizing how far they'd come in their own knowledge and healing, and knowing that what they'd learned could help others they cared about.

They decided to hold monthly living-room meetings with friends, coworkers, and acquaintances to share their newfound knowledge. Week by week, more people found their way to these meetings, and soon there was quite a crowd.

Over time, they had attracted a group of dedicated healers and practitioners, including doctors, who were able to help them to understand more and to keep improving their delivery of information. Everyone learned something. Soon a circle of dedicated leaders spread out to educate others, allowing these events to occur in different parts of the country, where people could learn more about how to stay well, while tackling whatever environmental situations contributed to the problem. As it grew, the Internet provided a mechanism for the Canary Club to spread new ideas and research as well as helping those affected to feel connected and to gain political power.

Meredith Enters a New Phase

Meredith had comfortably resolved her sex-hormone issues, leaving her much more focused and on target in her life. She now had plenty of time to devote to these groups, as her children were currently away at college. Once the fuzzy thinking was resolved, she began to take a closer look at her secondary challenge. While it wasn't bothering her anywhere near as much as the primary challenge had, she saw room for improvement and wanted to tackle this next gland, as well.

For Meredith, this perimenopausal stage put additional pressure on her thyroid system. No matter how well balanced the female hormones may be, when a woman goes through menopause, there are increased demands for the thyroid to handle the dynamics of change.

Many women who are approaching or are in menopause and whose thyroid was reasonably balanced previously now experience low-thyroid symptoms. Their gland is not able to keep up with the increased output of thyroid hormone required. A similar change occurs at puberty. A child with a tendency for low thyroid can be sufficiently compensated and thereby adequately balanced thyroidwise in the early years of life. But with the change of puberty comes additional demands for thyroid hormone, which results in a previously borderline situation now becoming frankly hypothyroid. The teenager may gain weight, develop terrible acne, start suffering in school due to sluggish mental function.

Both the pubescent teen and the menopausal mom may need extra thyroid support measures for a year or two during these times of transition. What did this mean for Meredith?

She found herself having more sluggish bowel function. She increased her fiber and drank more water, which was helpful. Her memory was still fine, but now she experienced accelerated hair loss and the annoyance of cracking, peeling nails. Her skin became so dry that she seemingly spent hours daily either scratching or applying creams. The last straw was when her tongue seemed to be getting too large for her mouth, causing her to bite it frequently.

Recognizing these as possible thyroid symptoms, she took the home testing by both blood spot and saliva. Sure enough, her TSH was now much higher than it had been previously, and her Free T4 and Free T3 were too low.

This indicated hypothyroidism, so she embarked upon the home remedy program suggested in chapter 6 for low thyroid. After a couple of months of being very diligent, she found that she was not improving as quickly as she wanted, so she sought medical support. She took her test results and symptom list to her doctor, who suggested that it was time for a trial of prescription thyroid medicine. She was put on one grain of natural thyroid, as she preferred using natural treatments instead of synthetic ones whenever possible.

The results were dramatic. In less than two weeks, her skin condition

cleared up by 90 percent, and her tongue became more normal. In an-
other two weeks, the hair loss had slowed to a more acceptable rate.
Best of all, she no longer needed extra fiber and tons of water to have
better intestinal regularity. For her, the thyroid prescription involved a
daily pill for the better part of a year. She then weaned off the prescrip-
tion medicine and continued with only the nonprescription thyroid
boosters.

Meredith's story illustrates that timing is everything. She did not need **physical** endo-type intervention before the onset of perimenopause. If she had tried it, it may have complicated her situation. She did not need thyroid intervention after this perimenopause time. But she did need it during perimenopause, specifically.

Many people go through a critical period where hormonal support is needed for a short time, not forever. To know when that crucial moment is upon us, and to take advantage of it, is what brings you the greatest benefit.

Also, to know what type of action you need to take is equally important. Being able to reassess your three major energy hormones at various times in your life will help you update your road map as needed.

Phoebe

Phoebe was sailing along, feeling great. She ended up not needing to make any further changes and has continued to do very well, even without prescription medicine.

Emily's Path

Emily was a different story. Once she had her adrenal system more in balance, she was a whole new person, more like her old self. Her friends again referred to her as the perennial happy camper. She had recently married. The stock business had its usual ups and downs, but she man-aged to prosper and gain the respect of her employees at work.

The only challenge occurred several years later. While her adrenal system seemed to recover nicely, and she did not have thyroid symp-toms, she began to have very difficult PMS. This started innocently enough with her feeling under the weather for a day or two before each period. It grew in severity and duration so that before long she was having two full weeks of very uncomfortable breast tenderness, bloating and actual swelling of fingers and ankles several days prior to her period. Emily took her questionnaires again, as well as the home tests. They all pointed to estrogen dominance (progesterone deficiency). She received some benefit from estrogen reduction maneuvers outlined in chapter 7, but was only fully back to normal when she added twice-daily applications of progesterone cream.

The over-the-counter version worked passably well, but she found even greater benefit from a stronger, more potent cream prescribed by her doctor, made up personally for her by a local compounding pharmacy.

This worked perfectly until her periods ceased at menopause. Just as happened with Meredith, the transition into menopause put enormous strain on her glandular system. Perhaps the same reason her adrenal glands had been low when she was younger was now, at this age, causing other glands to suffer. This is what can happen when the autoimmune phenomenon, quite common as a genetic predisposition, is triggered by major life changes.

Her testing showed high levels of thyroid antibodies, indicating that now a thyroid version of the autoimmune tendency was currently becoming symptomatic. She handled this thyroid problem with her practitioner's prescription for synthetic thyroxine. After two years on this regimen, she was able to wean off slowly. Since then, as long as she adheres to her natural protocols, she feels fine.

Emily's long-term progression illustrates how one person can go through all three endo-types at different times of her life. Some people are not as fortunate as Emily. They have all three endo-types in a much more compacted fashion, one right after the other and in rapid fire. In fact, some people experience all three endo-typical situations simultaneously.

Once again, the best evaluation for all three of these challenges is to fill out the questionnaires and perform home testing then to identify which gland is the *major culprit* at any one moment. Intervening on that prime issue first then seeing how much benefit is available before intervening on the others generally leads to a more satisfactory result.

Once the primary situation has been handled adequately, attention can then be diverted to the secondary challenge, if necessary at that particular time. Then, and only then, might someone choose to focus on a tertiary challenge.

It is possible that one would need to continue the treatments of the primary and secondary problems, and perhaps even address the tertiary one, simultaneously. This can be confusing, and requires considerable skill on the part of the practitioner and dedication on the part of the patient. When such intervention is required, it can bring much-needed relief.

Generally, whenever possible, the best approach is to focus on one challenge at a time, perhaps for a period of months, or even seasons of the year, before adding interventions for the secondary or tertiary challenges.

The Canary Chorus

How did things turn out for our three women and their desire to spread the word about hormonal balance? Their respective health and vitality allowed them to devote sufficient time and energy to help create what they hoped would become an important social contribution. They coined it the Canary Club.

They joined forces and helped to create a Web site (www.canary club.org) to support those who want to hear from knowledgeable practitioners, and to compare notes and discuss their lives with those similarly challenged. It was growing into a phenomenon that seemed to have a life of its own.

Neither Emily, Phoebe, nor Meredith wanted to run this themselves. In fact, they felt that there should not really be any leader or boss. Instead, they gave everyone they spoke to the advice that each local Canary Club chapter should be autonomous and self-directing, perhaps having occasional meetings in various members' living rooms, similar to the way Weight Watchers and Alcoholics Anonymous had gotten started. They feel, and we agree, that autoimmune glandular illness may affect 40 million people in the United States alone. It is clearly a worldwide and growing problem, one that deserves to be a larger part of our society's health care dialogue.

We look forward to a new dawn, a time of reflection and realization, a time to inspire the joining of hearts and minds for a healthier tomorrow. You may feel fat, fuzzy, or frazzled today, but take heart, and join the chorus. Tomorrow you could be a Canary Club leader, feeling fit, focused, and fabulous.

FEELING FIT, FOCUSED, AND FABULOUS!

As we promised at the start of this program, having a level and solid three-legged stool can be one of life's surprisingly great joys. With this secure metabolic foundation to build upon, everything else in your life can go better.

Weight-loss efforts now work readily, and the results are long-lasting. Memory and concentration are much more dependable, at your command, and effective for achieving your goals. Most welcome, however, is the ability to live in greater peace and harmony, within yourself and among others.

We sincerely hope this has been a deeply rewarding journey. May your benefits continue to multiply, using this book as your road map, so that you can become the person you have always wanted to be, attracting your highest visions while living your most fabulous life.

Keep enjoying the ride!

APPENDICES

Many of the products mentioned in the Appendix may be ordered from www.FeelingFFF.com or by calling (866) 468-4979.

AUTHORS' NOTE: While we have made every effort to provide accurate telephone numbers, mailing addresses, Internet addresses, and product information, the information provided herein may change after this writing. The authors maintain business relationships with several of the suppliers whose products are mentioned in the following pages.

ORDERING YOUR HOME LAB TESTS

DIAGNOS-TECHS

Diagnos-Techs, Inc.
www.diagnostechs.com
6620 South 192nd Place, Building J
Kent, WA 98032
Phone: (800) 878-3787
Fax: (425) 251-0637

Diagnos-Techs, Inc., was established in 1987 and was the first lab in the United States to implement salivary-based hormone assessment into routine clinical practice. For the past twelve years, their tests have converted many physicians in their hormone assay preferences from run-of-the-mill mass-production blood panels to precision diagnosis of problems. These tests have become powerful tools in evaluating gastrointestinal problems, stress- and hormone-related diseases, and overall wellness. Quality control is clearly a primary goal. All parameters on reports are standardized daily to WHO (World Health Organization) and other standardization agencies' reference materials. This ensures the reproducibility of results and permits precise clinical diagnosis based on real values, year in and year out.

You can secure high-quality home testing at low cost through a new patient advocacy group called the Canary Club, to which we are the medical advisors. To enroll in this organization, you sign up on line at www.canary club.org, enabling you to order and obtain reduced-fee testing under the umbrella of the organization. Upon joining, you will be supplied with a password and code number that enables you to place your order directly with the lab. Diagnos-Techs can also help with physician referrals for knowledgeable practitioners in your locale.

Special Note

While all the labs listed are excellent and provide similar testing, only Diagnos-Techs will allow you as a consumer to order testing without a private practitioner and receive the results directly. At the time of this writing, Diagnos-Techs is donating a small portion of their fee for club expenses and scholarships.

The Canary Club Panel of simplified testing includes the following items:

- Thyroid Saliva Panel: The main components of a full thyroid evaluation generally done on blood samples are now available to be checked via a one-sample saliva determination.
- Adrenal Stress Index: This involves four separate samples of saliva for cortisol and DHEA collected at four different times during the day.
- Reproductive Hormone Screen: This is a one-time saliva determination for a quick check of the major reproductive hormones in both men and women (estrogen and progesterone for women, testosterone for men).

Complete directions for all testing and panels come with the sample collection kit, which is mailed to you by the lab (unless your personal practitioner already has them in her or his office). Results of testing will be mailed directly to you to help you determine your actual endo-type (see chapter 4). Once again, we urge you to review these results with a supportive and knowledgeable practitioner of your choice.

ZRT LABORATORY

1815 NW 169th Place, Suite 5050
Beaverton, OR 97006.
Phone: (503) 466-2445
Fax: (503) 466-1636
www.salivatest.com, www.bloodspottest.com
Hormone Hotline: (503) 466-9166

The Hormone Hotline is a twenty-four-hour taped audio-library with a growing list of topics on every aspect of hormone balance and testing.

ZRT Laboratory is a CLIA certified hormone-testing laboratory in Beaverton, Oregon. It was established in 1998 and is independently owned and operated by David T. Zava, PhD, a biochemist and breast-cancer researcher. ZRT Laboratory developed cutting-edge technology for saliva and blood spot sample processing and analysis. It is the only large-volume clinical laboratory to remove contaminants that may alter test results. Using advanced methods of testing, ZRT's hormone evaluation can help identify preventable hormone imbalances that may be causing symptoms associated with chronic disease and rapid aging. In addition, ZRT is the only large-scale laboratory that documents and monitors patient-reported symptoms and relates these back to tested hormone levels.

Complete directions for home sample collection of individual hormones and panels come with the test kit, which is mailed to you by the lab unless your practitioner already has them in her or his office. ZRT Lab uses a finger-prick blood-spot test rather than saliva for thyroid evaluations.

Testing at this lab must be ordered by a licensed health-care provider.

GREAT SMOKIES DIAGNOSTIC LABORATORY
63 Zillicoa Street
Asheville, NC 28801
Phone: (800) 522-4762
www.gsdl.com

Call to inquire about the types of testing offered, and to access the physician-referral service to find a physician near you. These tests must be ordered by a licensed health care provider.

Established in 1986, Great Smokies Diagnostic Laboratory has helped pioneer the field of laboratory functional testing. Functional testing assesses the dynamic interrelationship of physiological systems, thereby creating a more complete picture of one's health, unlike traditional allopathic testing, which is more concerned about the pathology of disease. By supporting the practitioner in identifying the root cause of chronic conditions, functional testing helps the practitioner to develop optimal interventions to assist patients in their quest for achieving lasting health.

This laboratory serves over eight thousand primary and specialty physicians and health-care providers worldwide, offering over 125 specialized diagnostic assessments. These innovative tests cover a wide range of physiological areas, including digestive, immune, nutritional, endocrine, metabolic function—along with GENOVATIONS profiles targeting modifiable effects of gene polymorphism. The laboratory is accredited by the College of American Pathologists and fully licensed by HCFA.

BIOHEALTH LABORATORIES
BioHealth Diagnostics
2929 Canon Street
San Diego, CA 92106
Phone: (800) 570-2000
Fax: (800) 720-7239
www.biodia.com

BioHealth Diagnostics, headquartered in San Diego, California, was founded by Dr. William G. Timmins, ND, in 1998 to meet the needs of health care professionals seeking better solutions to their patients' health challenges. Dr. Timmins' experience working with chronically ill patients and training doctors led him to develop the finest in laboratory testing, nutritional supplementation, treatment programs, physician training, and patient health education. BioHealth Diagnostics Laboratories, located in Santa Monica, California, is headquarters for research and development projects. This facility is responsible for turning the specimens of patients everywhere into accurate, objective laboratory reports.

Complete directions for all testing and panels come with the sample collection kit, which is mailed to you by the lab unless your practitioner already has them in her or his office.

Testing at this lab must be ordered by a licensed health-care provider.

For More Information
For those interested in reviewing research on the validity of home saliva testing, we recommend the following articles and Web site as a beginning:

- "Salivary Steroid Assays for Assessing Variation in Endocrine Activity" Authors: D. Riad-Fahmy, G. F. Read, and R. F. Walker. Facility: Tenovus Institute for Cancer Research, Welsh National School of Medicine, Heath Park, Cardiff, Wales.
- "The Measurement of Hormones in Saliva: Possibilities and Pitfalls" Authors: Ross F. Vining and Robynne A. McGinley. Facility: Garvan Institute of Medical Research, St. Vincent's Hospital, Sydney, Australia.
- "Assessing Estradiol in Biobehavioral Studies Using Saliva and Blood Spots: Simple Radioimmunoassay Protocols, Reliability and Comparative Validity" Authors: Elizabeth A. Shirtcliff, et al. Facility: Behavioral Endocrinology Laboratory, Dept of Biobehavioral Health, Pennsylvania State University.

- Salimetrics, State College, Pennsylvania; Department of Sociology, Pennsylvania State University; Psychology Department, University of North Carolina at Wilmington.
- Also you will find an extensive research section called "Saliva Reference Summary" at www.salivatest.com.

LOCATING YOUR RECOMMENDED VITAMINS

There are thousands of companies and products related to the issues presented in this book. *For the purposes of ensuring that you get the best possible start,* we are recommending initially only those top organizations run by people we have personally met, whose work we highly respect, and whose product formulas are ideally suited to gland rebalancing. As you improve, you can explore other options should you so desire. Since many readers are stressed and busy, we are making our simplest yet best suggestions for immediate results.

Please read through the various descriptions and feel free to contact the companies for further information. They will provide excellent support in helping you to choose the best products for your endo-type and budget.

XYMOGEN

Xymogen has more than twenty-five years of experience, operating as Atlantic ProNutrients or APN, in providing exclusive professional formulas to healthcare practitioners. (Readers of this book may order directly by mentioning Dr. Shames.) As an independent health sciences company, Xymogen has introduced numerous innovations to the functional medicine community.

The Xymogen line of formulas was researched and developed based on the overwhelming demands of their customers, with regard to maintaining the most effective nutraceuticals on the market.

To reach Xymogen, call (800) 647-6100. Mention Dr. Shames when ordering and you may be eligible for a discount.

General Formulas—
A Four-Product Program for All Endo-Types:
- **Active Nutrients** (basic multivitamin-multimineral)
  A balanced formula containing vitamins, minerals, and trace elements, serves as an excellent multivitamin and multimineral for general nutri-

tional support. The ingredients are in the form most conducive to maximal absorption and utilization in the body.

- **Oraxinol** (a full-potency antioxidant)
  This is an innovative blend of standardized formulas that have a very high ORAC (oxygen radical absorption capacity), a measurement of antioxidants found in fruits and vegetables. This helps to minimize the effects of free radicals on the aging process.

- **OmegaPure EFA** (crucial fatty acids)
  Combining alpha-linolenic acid (omega-3) and linoleic acid (omega-6), this product is exceptionally beneficial as an essential fatty acid formula. This is one of the few products to combine fish, flax, and borage oils as rich sources of necessary ingredients for maintaining cell membrane integrity and immune function.

- **IgG Pure** (aminos and protein for immune balance)
  A patented and ultrafiltered whey protein concentrate with a standardized source of immunoglobulins obtained from New Zealand herds (free from environmental contaminants). It has been proved in clinical trials to stimulate the immune system, fight pathogens, and promote the development of lean body mass.

Specific Additional Products for Your Individual Endo-Type:

- **MedCaps T3** (for **physical** endo-types)
  Features targeted nutrients and herbs that support healthy thyroid hormone synthesis. The herbal combination of ashwagandha and guggul aids in the conversion of T4 to T3 and may facilitate the expression of thyroid hormone genes. An exceptional thyroid product.

- **MedCaps PMS** (for **mental** endo-types—menstruating women)
  An ideal formula for the premenopausal woman, this product contains a unique blend of vitamins and herbs to support women with symptoms associated with their menstrual cycle. It assists the liver in hormone metabolism and balance, as well as supporting muscular function.

- **MedCaps Menopause** (for **mental** endo-types—nonmenstruating women)
  A unique combination formulated to provide targeted biochemical nourishment for women during menopause and beyond. It features selected herbs and non–soy derived nutrients that support the body's

adaptive response, as well as supporting circulation, relaxation, and overall well-being.

- **Viriligen** (for **mental** endo-types—men)
An all-natural sexual enhancer, featuring a proprietary blend of herbs that support men in healthy sexual function and hormone balance. Horny goat weed, yanhusuo, and yohimbe combine to enhance levels of dopamine, testosterone metabolism, and blood flow.

- **Adrenal Essence** (for **emotional** endo-types)
One of the most useful of all adrenal supports, this product helps to reduce negative effects of stress and fatigue. This formula is ideal for those who lead stressful lives, or who are constantly exposed to elevated stress hormones and the accompanying exhaustion. Three different herbal adaptogens and specific adrenal vitamins combine to help return the body back to balance and more optimal function.

METAGENICS

Metagenics is one of the nation's largest sponsors of continuing education for health practitioners. Its exclusive formulas are generally only available through professional providers, so readers of this book may order directly by mentioning Dr. Shames.

The company was founded in 1983 with the mission to improve health by helping people achieve their genetic potential through nutrition. The company is headquartered in San Clemente, California, with its world-class Functional Medicine Research Center (FMRC) and manufacturing facility located in Gig Harbor, Washington.

To order products and to learn more about Metagenics, visit www .feelingfff.com.

General Formulas—
A Four-Product Program for All Endo-Types:

- **MultiGenics** (multivitamin with minerals)
Multigenics is a comprehensive multiple vitamin and mineral formula suitable for adolescents, adults, and seniors that provides an essential, comprehensive foundation for optimal health (seniors and nonmenstruating women should choose Multigenics without Iron).

- **Oxygenics** (a full-symphony antioxidant)
Oxygenics is a superb formula comprising a comprehensive blend of antioxidants and precursor nutrients to support antioxidant systems within the body. This formula may help protect against most

categories of free radicals such as superoxide, hydrogen peroxide, hydroxyl, peroxyl, hypochlorite, and singlet oxygen.

- **Omega-EFA** (balanced fatty acids)
  Omega-EFA is a specially balanced blend of the essential fatty acids EPA, DHA, and GLA. It supports a healthy balance of eicosanoids— a group of hormonelike compounds produced in the body. A healthy balance of eicosanoids supports proper cardiovascular, nervous, and immune system function.

- **BioPure Protein** (amino acids and immunoglobulins)
  Amino acids are important for lean muscle tissue, endurance, and hormone production. Because humans lack the ability to synthesize certain amino acids, these are referred to as essential amino acids. BioPure Protein is a bioactive amino acid source with naturally occurring immunoglobulins (antibodies), which promote immune system activity.

Specific Additional Products for Your Individual Endo-Type:

- **Thyrosol** (for **physical** endo-types)
  Recommended for men and women of **physical** endo-type. Thyrosol is an exciting multifaceted formula featuring targeted nutrients and herbs that promote healthy thyroid function. Many aspects of health, including body composition and energy level are impacted by thyroid hormone activity.

- **EstroFactors** (for **mental** endo-types—women)
  EstroFactors promotes healthy hormone balance in women of all ages by featuring targeted nutrients that support healthy estrogen metabolism and detoxification. Supporting a healthy balance of hormones may provide significant relief for women with hormone-related health issues. In particular, soy isoflavones, folic acid, indole-3-carbinol, black cohosh, chasteberry, dong quai, ginseng, and vitamin B_6, B_{12}, and E may be beneficial for women seeking a safe and natural way to maintain their hormonal health.

- **Ultra Prostagen** (for **mental** endo-types—men)
  Combinations of select herbs, amino acids, and nutrients have been designed to support prostate health, proper urination, and male vitality and stamina. Ultra Prostagen is a blend of raw prostate concentrate with saw palmetto, pumpkin seed, amino acids, zinc, and other select nutrients in a formula designed specially for men.

- **Mentalin** (for **mental** endo-types—men and women)

An excellent brain-support formula that combines traditionally used herbal extracts to enhance mental function, alertness, and memory. The herbs are provided in a standard extract of bacopa and gotu kola as well as supportive amounts of a dozen other highly recommended ayurvedic herbs.

- **Licorice Plus** (for **emotional** endo-types)
  This is a specially designed herbal adrenal support that combines standardized extracts of licorice, ashwagandha, rehmannia, and Chinese yam. Its unparalleled action of licorice in association with exceptional adaptogens is recommended for early stages of adrenal challenge. (People with high blood pressure must use this product cautiously.)
- **Adrenogen** (raw glandular concentrate for **emotional** endo-types)
  The body's adrenal glands produce stress hormones, steroid hormones, and blood pressure–regulating hormones. Adrenogen, useful for **emotional** endo-types, provides nutritional support for adrenal function by combining high-quality nutrients that are involved in hormone regulation.

OTHER EXCELLENT COMPANIES WHOSE PRODUCTS WE PERSONALLY RECOMMEND AND HIGHLY ENDORSE

You can access more information about other fine companies by going to **www.FeelingFFF.com**. There we have listed these several additional companies with our specific endo-type recommendations for many of their products.

NEW SPIRIT NATURALS

The founders of New Spirit, Dr. Larry and Debbie Milam, are innovative pioneers whose uniquely formulated products are distributed worldwide due to their exceptional efficacy.

Call (800) 922-2766 for customer service. Mention Dr. Shames and you may be eligible for a discount.

ECONUGENICS

The founder of EcoNugenics, Isaac Eliaz, MD, L.Ac., is a highly respected medical doctor and acupuncturist, who studied oriental medicine in the East and has been in practice for over twenty years. His advanced formulations are extremely creative and highly effective. EcoNugenics holds the U.S. patent on Padma Basic, an exceptional thyroid-boosting product.

Call (800) 308-5518 to order. Mention Dr. Shames and you may be eligible for a discount.

SUNRIDER INTERNATIONAL

Established in 1982, this innovative manufacturer offers food-grade system-specific healthy living products. Karilee has been taking several of these for many years with excellent results.

Toll-free USA: (800) 9-HERBS-9 (943-7279).
Outside USA: (760) 744-3477
Web site: Go to www.FeelingFFF.com.

LEGACY FOR LIFE

Legacy for Life was created in October 1998 to market and distribute the recent breakthroughs in hyperimmune egg technology for immune regulating and hormone balancing. The company employs the highest standards in bringing to market cutting-edge research. Their Immune 26 egg powder is highly restorative for all endo-types.

Call (800) 385-0584. Mention Dr. Shames when ordering and you may be eligible for a discount.
Fax: (305) 233-1149

WOBENZYM

Wobenzym is the world's most researched systemic enzyme formula. Millions of people around the world use it to activate a variety of healing processes to reduce gland inflammation that often results in glandular imbalance. Clinical studies have found that Wobenzym promotes robust circulation, a strong immune system, and healthy aging.

For those desiring this product mentioned in several places throughout this book, it can be ordered by calling EcoNugenics above.

FINAL THOUGHTS

In addition to the above companies, we highly recommend that, when you have time, you browse through your local health food stores and keep learning more about their products. There are many excellent health food and vitamin stores across the country that are serving people well by providing high-quality items and information to consumers. Many of these nondiscounted health food stores have excellent products. Locate one that has well-trained and educated staff that can help you.

FURTHER READING AND HORMONE RESEARCH

While there are literally thousands of books, and many thousands of research articles, on the topics mentioned in these twelve chapters, we have selected a representative list of books and papers that suggest some recent trends in current scientific thinking.

The hormone-related books are listed first, in alphabetical order by author, then a list of some current relevant research articles that we have found useful in guiding our program.

First, however, you may find it helpful to read a bit more of the Shames health approach, as explained in our prior books and articles (as listed below), and also be sure to visit **www.shameshealth.com.**

BOOKS BY KARILEE AND RICHARD SHAMES, MD

Shames, R. L. and Shames, K. H. *Thyroid Power: 10 Steps to Total Health.* NY: HarperResource, 2001 (hardcover) 2002 (paperback).

Shames, K. *Creative Imagery in Nursing.* Albany, NY: Delmar Publishers, 1996.

Shames, K. *The Nightingale Conspiracy.* Montclair, NJ: Enlightenment Press, 1993.

Shames, R. and Shames, K. *The Gift of Health.* New York: Bantam Books, 1982.

Shames, R. and Sterin, C. *Healing with Mind Power.* Emmaus, PA: Rodale Press, 1978.

Hover-Kramer, D. and Shames, K. *Energetic Approaches to Emotional Healing.* Albany, NY: Delmar Publishers, 1997.

ARTICLES BY AND INTERVIEWS WITH DRS. RICHARD AND KARILEE SHAMES (FULL TEXT AVAILABLE ON WWW.THYROIDPOWER.COM)

Autoimmune Hypothyroidism—A Mind-Body Exploration
The Adrenal–Thyroid Connection
Are Thyroid Cysts Normal?
Thyroid Related Hair Loss
Fluoride: A Bad Idea Whose Time Has Passed
Causes of an Underactive Thyroid
Breaking News: Estrogen, Menopause and Thyroid
The Thyroid/Menopause Connection
Thyroid Related Sex Drive Problems
What's the Best BRAND of Thyroid for Me?
Synthetic vs Natural Thyroid Drugs—Are Synthetic More Stable?
Optimal Synthroid-Cytomel Combination
When to Get a Second Opinion
Hypothyroidism Tests and Doctors
Can Basal Body Temperatures Diagnose Thyroid?
Saliva and Urine Tests for Thyroid Disease
Men versus Women with Thyroid Problems
Avoiding "Tyranny of the Test": Your Optimal Med Dose

HORMONE BALANCE–RELATED BOOKS

Ashford, N., Miller, C. *Chemical Exposures: Low Levels and High Stakes.* New York, NY: Van Nostrand Reinhold, 1998.

Ashner, L., Goldstein, S. R. *Could It Be . . . Perimenopause: How Women 35–50 Can Overcome Forgetfulness, Mood Swings, Insomnia, Weight Gain, Sexual Dysfunction and Other Telltale Signs of Hormonal Imbalance.* New York, NY: Little Brown, 2000.

Bryson, C. *The Fluoride Deception.* New York, NY: Seven Stories Press, 2004.

Carson, R. *Silent Spring.* New York, NY: Houghton Mifflin Company, 1962.

Colburn, T., et al. *Our Stolen Future: Are We Threatening Our Fertility, Intelligence, and Survival?* New York, NY: Dutton, 1996.

D'Adamo, P., Whitney, C. *Live Right for Your Type.* New York, NY: Putnam, 2001.

Dadd, D. L. *Home Safe Home: Protecting Yourself and Your Family from Everyday Toxics and Harmful Household Products in the Home.* Los Angeles, CA: Jeremy Tarcher, 1997.

Diamond, J. *The Whole Man Program: Reinvigorating Your Body, Mind, and Spirit After 40.* Hoboken, NJ: Wiley, 2003.

Fuchs, N. K. *Overcoming the Legacy of Overeating: How to Change Your Negative Eating Patterns,* Third Ed. Chicago, IL: Lowell House, 1999.

Gittleman, A. L., Greggains, J. *The Fat Flush Fitness Plan.* New York, NY: McGraw-Hill, 2003.

Haas, E. *The False Fat Diet: The Revolutionary 21 Day Program for Losing the Weight You Think Is Fat.* New York, NY: Ballantine Books, 2000.

Jefferies, W. *Safe Uses of Cortisone,* Second Ed. Springfield, IL: Charles C. Thomas Publishers, 1996.

Jordan, L.T. *Fat & Furious: A Look at Weight Loss Issues from the Mind-Body Perspective.* Campbell, CA: L. T. J. Associates, 2004.

Kidd, P. *Phosphatidyl Serine: The Nutrient Building Block That Accelerates All Brain Functions and Counters Alzheimer's Disease.* Los Angeles, CA: Keats Publishing, 1998.

Klaiber, E. L. *Hormones and the Mind: A Woman's Guide to Enhancing Mood, Memory, and Sexual Vitality.* New York, NY: Perennial Currents, 2002.

Krimsky, S. *Hormonal Chaos: The Scientific and Social Origins of the Environmental Endocrine Hypothesis.* Baltimore, MD: Johns Hopkins Press, 2000.

Kristal, H., Haig, J. *The Nutrition Solution: A Guide to Your Metabolic Type.* Berkeley, CA: North Atlantic Books, 2002.

Lee, J. *What Your Doctor May Not Tell You About Menopause.* New York, NY: Warner Books, 1996.

Lee, J. *What Your Doctor May Not Tell You About Premenopause.* New York, NY: Warner Books, 1999.

Pert, C. *Molecules of Emotion.* New York, NY: Scribner, 1997.

Ross, J. *The Diet Cure: An 8-Step Program to Rebalance Your Body Chemistry.* New York, NY: Viking, 1999.

Ross, J. *The Mood Cure: The 4-Step Program to Rebalance Your Emotional Chemistry and Rediscover Your Natural Sense of Well-Being.* New York, NY: Viking, 2002.

Rossman, M. *Healing Yourself: A Step by Step Program for Better Health Through Imagery.* New York, NY: Walker & Co., 1987.

Seaman, B. *The Greatest Experiment Ever Performed on Women.* New York, NY: Hyperion Books, 2003.

Selye, H. *The Stress of Life.* New York, NY: McGraw Hill, 1956.

Shomon, M. J. *Living Well with Hypothyroidism.* New York, NY: Avon Books, 2000.

Shomon, M. J. *Living Well with Autoimmune Disease: What Your Doctor Doesn't Tell You ... That You Need to Know*. New York, NY: HarperResource, 2002.

Shomon, M. J. *The Thyroid Diet: Manage Your Metabolism for Lasting Weight Loss*. New York, NY: HarperResource, 2004.

Sichel, D., Driscoll, J. W. *Women's Moods: What Every Woman Must Know About Hormones, the Brain, and Emotional Health*, First Quill edition. New York, NY: Perennial Currents, 2000.

Siegal, S. *Is Your Thyroid Making You Fat?* New York: Warner Books, 2000.

Somers, S. *The Sexy Years: Discover the Hormone Connection—The Secret to Fabulous Sex, Great Health, and Vitality for Women and Men*. New York, NY: Crown Publishers, 2004.

Steingraber, S. *Living Downstream*. New York, NY: Vintage Books, 1998.

Steinman, D., Epstein, S. *The Safe Shopper's Bible: A Consumer's Guide to Nontoxic Household Products*. New York, NY: Ceres Press, 1994.

Vliet, E. *Women, Weight and Hormones*. New York, NY: M. Evans, 2001.

Volpe, R. *Autoimmunity in Endocrine Diseases*. Boca Raton, FL: CRC Press, 1990.

Warga, C. L. *Menopause and the Mind: The Complete Guide to Coping with Memory Loss, Foggy Thinking, Verbal Confusion, and Other Cognitive Effects of Perimenopause and Menopause*. New York, NY: Simon & Schuster, 1999.

Wargo, J. *Our Children's Toxic Legacy: How Science and Law Fail to Protect Us from Pesticides*. New Haven, CT: Yale University Press, 1998.

Wilson, J. L. *Adrenal Fatigue: The 21st-Century Stress Syndrome*. Petaluma, CA: Smart Publications, 2002.

Zimmerman, S. *My Doctor Says I'm Fine ... So Why Do I Feel So Bad?* Nevada City, CA: Blue Dolphin Publishing, 2001.

Research Articles Related to Integrative Hormone Balance

Aleman A., Bronk E., Kessels R. P., Koppeschaar H. P., van Honk, J. "A single administration of testosterone improves visuospatial ability in young women." *Psychoneuroendocrinology*. Jun 2004; 29(5):612–7.

Arlt W., Callies F., van Vlijmen J. C., et al. "DHEA replacement in women with adrenal insufficiency." *N Engl J Med*. Sep 30 1999; 341(14): 1013–20.

Azad N., Pitale S., Barnes W. E., Friedman N. "Testosterone treatment enhances regional brain perfusion in hypogonadal men." *J Clin Endocrinol Metab*. Jul 2003; 88(7):3064–8.

Becker, N., et al. "The APICH syndrome (allergy-polyendocrine-immunity-candida hypersensivity)." *Western Med.* 145: 388–91 (1986).

Bjorntorp PA. "Overweight is risking fate." *Baillieres Best Pract Res Clin Endocrinol Metab.* Apr 1999; 13(1):47–69.

Cherrier M. M., Craft S., Matsumoto A. H. "Cognitive changes associated with supplementation of testosterone or dihydrotestosterone in mildly hypogonadal men: a preliminary report." *J Androl.* Jul–Aug 2003; 24(4):568–76.

Christiansen J. J., Gravholt C. H., Fisker S., et al. "Dehydroepiandrosterone (DHEA) supplementation in women with adrenal failure: impact on twenty-four-hour GH secretion and IGF-related parameters." *Clin Endocrinol.* (Oxford, England). Apr 2004; 60(4): 461–9.

Fedotova Y. O. "The effects of the hormones of peripheral endocrine glands on the processes of behavior, learning, and memory." *Neurosci Behav Physiol.* Jan–Feb 2000; 30(1): 75–80.

Fraser, W. et al. "Are biochemical (blood) tests of thyroid function of any value in monitoring patients receiving thyroxine replacement?" *Br Med J* (Clin Res Ed). Sep 1986; 293(6550): 808–10.

Gambineri A., Pelusi C., Vicennati V., Pagotto U., Pasquali R. "Obesity and the polycystic ovary syndrome." *Int J Obes Relat Metab Disord.* Jul 2002; 26(7):883–96.

Gillett M. J., Martins R. N., Clarnette R. M., Chubb S. A., Bruce D. G., Yeap B. B. "Relationship between testosterone, sex hormone-binding globulin and plasma amyloid beta peptide 40 in older men with subjective memory loss or dementia." *J Alzheimers Dis.* Aug 2003; 5(4):267–9

Hautanen A. "Synthesis and regulation of sex hormone-binding globulin in obesity." *Int J Obes Relat Metab Disord* (England). Jun 2000; 24 (Suppl 2): S64–70.

Heim C., Ehlert U., Hellhammer D. H. "The potential role of hypocortisolism in the pathophysiology of stress-related bodily disorders." *Psychoneuroendocrinology* (England). Jan 2000; 25(1): 1–35.

Hogervorst E., Combrinck M., Smith A. D. "Testosterone and gonadotropin levels in men with dementia." *Neuro Endocrinol Lett.* Jun–Aug 2003; 24(3–4):203–8.

Hogervorst E., De Jager C., Budge M., Smith A. D. Abstract. "Serum levels of estradiol and testosterone and performance in different cognitive domains in healthy elderly men and women." *Psychoneuroendocrinology.* Apr 2004; 29(3):405–21.

Kasperlik-Zaluska, A. "High prevalence of thyroid autoimmunity in idiopathic Addison's disease." *Autoimmunity.* 1994; 18(3): 213–6.

Keefe D. L. "Sex hormones and neural mechanisms." *Arch Sex Behav.* Oct 2002; 31(5): 401–6.

Kendler B. S. "Nutritional endocrinology." *Nutrition.* Jan 2003; 19(1):86–9.

Langley K., Hepp R., Grant N. J., et al. "Thyroid hormones regulate adrenal chromaffin cell SNAP-25." *Ann NY Acad Sci.* Oct 2002; (971): 277–80.

Maheu F. S., Lupien S. J. Review. "Memory in the grip of emotions and stress: a necessarily harmful impact?" *Med Sci* (Paris). Jan 2003; 19(1):118–24.

Meckling K. A., O'Sullivan C., Saari D. "Comparison of a low-fat diet to a low-carbohydrate diet on weight loss, body composition, and risk factors for diabetes and cardiovascular disease in free-living, overweight men and women." *J Clin Endocrinol Melab.* Jun 2004; 89 (6):2717–23.

Nilsson R. "Endocrine modulators in the food chain and environment." *Toxicol Pathol.* May–Jun 2000; 28(3):420–31.

Oelkers W., Diederich S., Bahr V. "Therapeutic strategies in adrenal insufficiency." *Ann Endocrinol* (Paris). Apr 2001; 62(2):212–6.

Robaczyk M. G. "Evaluation of leptin levels in plasma and their reliance on other hormonal factors affecting tissue fat levels in people with various levels of endogenous cortisol." *Ann Acad Med Stetin.* 2002; 48:283–300.

Toni R., Malaguti A., Castorina S., Roti E., Lechan R. M. "New paradigms in neuroendocrinology: relationships between obesity, systemic inflammation and the neuroendocrine system." *J Endocrinol Invest.* Feb 2004; 27(2):182–6.

Tsigos C., Chrousos G. P. "Hypothalamic-pituitary-adrenal axis, neuroendocrine factors and stress." *J Psychosom Res* (England). Oct 2002; 53(4): 865–71.

Wauters M., Considine R. V., Van Gaal L. F. "Human leptin: from an adipocyte hormone to an endocrine mediator." *Eur J Endocrinol* (England). Sep 2000; 143(3): 293–311.

FOR MORE INFORMATION

In this section, you will find Web sites and some phone numbers for organizations that can offer you further information and support, as well as help in finding personal practitioners in your area. Please note that this list is provided *in addition* to our favorite labs and vitamin companies mentioned earlier.

You can also contact Drs. Richard and Karilee Shames to learn more about their personalized hormonal telephone coaching service, that might include individual advice on tests, interpretation, and remedies.

Drs. Karilee and Richard Shames
www.FeelingFFF.com
(866) 468-4979
www.shameshealth.com and **www.thyroidpower.com**

HELPFUL WEB SITES

Related Information

www.canaryclub.com To become a member of the online community, the Canary Club. Provides related information, chat rooms, and online newsletters as well as resources and consumer advocacy to inspire better care for hormone challenges.

www.thyroid-info.com Consumer Advocate Mary Shomon's very detailed and well-researched site—wide-ranging and very helpful. Also has an excellent newsletter.

www.fluoridealert.org Fluoride Action Networks' Prolific source of antifluoride research and information. Home page contains excellent article by Dr. J. William Hirzy on "Why EPA's Headquarters Professionals' Union Opposes Fluoridation." A must-read for anyone concerned about health.

www.accessone.com/~watoxics Information clearinghouse and referral center promoting alternatives to toxic chemicals

www.wwfcanada.org/hormone-disruptors Endocrine disruptors

www.power-surge.com Selected as *Forbes* Best of the Web in 2001. One of the top sites for women looking for support and education during a turning point in their lives, menopause.

www.drlark.com Dr. Susan Lark Newsletter and Web site, very helpful for women

www.womenshealthletter.com Dr. Nan Kathryn Fuchs' newsletter and website for cutting-edge information on women's health issues. Excellent resource.

www.monitor.net/Rachel/ Update and dangers of toxic and endocrine-disrupting chemicals

Finding Practitioners

www.aanc.net The American Association of Nutritional Consultants offers an online directory of certified clinical nutritionists by last name, city, or state.

www.are-cayce.com Association for Research and Enlightenment Headquarters in Virginia Beach, VA

www.holisticmedicine.org American Holistic Medical Association (AHMA)

www.ahna.org American Holistic Nurses Association (AHNA)

www.acatoday.com The American Chiropractic Association (ACA)

www.aoa-net.org The American Osteopathic Association (AOA) offers an array of professional and personal benefits which provide support to osteopathic physicians and to the osteopathic profession.

www.acuall.org Web site for National Acupuncture and Oriental Medicine Alliance, providing referrals to practitioners in your area, as well as other information on the topic. They can be reached at (253) 851-6883.

www.bioset-institute.org Site for BioSet information, enzyme therapies by chiropractor and MD Ellen Cutler. Offers information and professional seminars.

info@amtamassage.org American Massage Therapy Association (AMTA)

www.abmp.com America Bodywork and Massage Professionals

www.hellerwork.com Hellerwork Association

www.rolf.org Rolfing Association

www.aston-patterning.com Aston/Patterning Association

www.imagroup.com International Aromatherapy Association

www.holisticmed.com General holistic site

www.homeopathyhome.com Homeopathy information

www.bloodph.com Personalized metabolic nutrition Web site, metabolic typing

www.extendedyears.com

www.naturopathic.org The American Association of Naturopathic Physicians Web site offers resources and information regarding disease prevention and health restoration. Most NPs use saliva testing.

www.bachflower.com Bach Flower Association

www.iacprx.org The International Academy of Compounding Pharmacists (IACP) an international, nonprofit association protecting and promoting the art and skill of pharmaceutical compounding. IACP's membership consists of more than 1,300 pharmacists who are committed to protecting the birthright of the profession of pharmacy-compounding.

www.pccarx.com Professional Compounding Centers of America. Excellent compounding pharmacist organization.

Water Filtration Devices

There are a variety of good companies offering filtration devices for your home or office. A good carbon block filter can eliminate many chemicals, including chlorine. To eliminate fluoride, you need a reverse-osmosis or a distillation device. Our favorite company for filters that could also give you further information is listed below.

Multi-Pure Corporation
Las Vegas Technology Center
P.O. Box 34630
Las Vegas, NV, 89133-4630
(800) 622-9206

You can also go to **www.nsf.gov** for a governmental rating of filtration devices.

Home Exercise Items

Our favorite piece of equipment is a small folding rebounder trampoline called the Cellerciser. (see **www.lightstreamers.com/CELLERCISER.htm**)

Thermometers for Basal Temperature Test

We recommend a nondigital basal thermometer for your home testing. The Geratherm Company of Switzerland makes an excellent one, sold in the United States by Longs Drug Stores and other pharmacy chains.

FINDING APPROPRIATE PRACTITIONERS

Part of being proactive about your health is making sure you are working with good practitioners, experienced in an open-minded and interactive manner, and willing to consider your input very carefully. To that end, we have considered all three endo-types below in terms of how they may relate to doctors based on their symptoms and related behaviors. This may help you to understand a little more about how to initiate the process of improving your doctor–patient relationship.

Physical endo-types often get into trouble when they see their gynecologist for a checkup and then allow him or her to prescribe sex hormones without testing. You will not be in a position to recover fully unless you are being treated appropriately. Remember, it is extremely difficult to balance your reproductive hormones when your thyroid is out of balance. In fact, it would be much like trying to use the rudder on a boat when the boat is standing still. This can feel like an exercise in futility, leading to years of disappointment and frustration. If your major endo-type is thyroid-driven, we strongly recommend that you balance the thyroid before initiating any program involving sex-hormone therapies.

Consider an endocrinologist at a university medical center, or a naturopathic doctor down the street; a family nurse practitioner or an acupuncturist with a special interest in gland balance. Laws vary from state to state, but many of these professionals can order testing and prescription medicines, should either of those be needed. Some alternative practitioners work in tandem with MDs in order to provide more comprehensive care. You may also choose to see practitioners who will make dietary and natural interventions prior to trying the more drastic prescription medicine that could further cloud the picture.

Emotional endo-types may not want to see an endocrinologist initially, as most are focused largely on diabetes, due to its epidemic proportions. If endocrinologists do devote time to adrenal balancing, it is generally to rule out Addison's or Cushing's diseases, the two most severe forms of low and high adrenal respectively. These doctors are not often aware of the subtle level of adrenal care that may be helpful to you. They are likely to do extensive blood testing and find nothing "wrong." More appropriate for your mild metabolic situation may be a naturopathic doctor, a well-trained holistic practitioner, a good nurse practitioner, or perhaps a physician assistant.

Adrenal-driven endo-types frequently are frazzled, don't sleep well, and can be irritable and nervous. As such, you should seek practitioners who can be calming and supportive, knowledgeable about specific ways to work with adrenal burnout, even in its earliest stages, helping to guide you to local services and resources for self-healing.

If you fall into the "fuzzy" sex gland–driven **mental** endo-type, you may be seeing a gynecologist. Keep in mind that most of these doctors are surgeons. In our opinion, the surgical mentality tends toward linear thinking, rather than having an open mind regarding a variety of interventions. The standard gynecologic approach may help with immediate symptom relief, but it can confuse the longer-term underlying issues. A "fuzzy" person might easily defer to the doctor, falling prey to an authority whose initial response would be to give something akin to a modern DES Band-Aid. In fact, in recent decades, millions of women have been encouraged to take Premarin and other heavy estrogenic compounds. Statistics have shown that many are later diagnosed with cancer. To us, it is like using a sledgehammer to open a peanut—it may not be the ideal first approach.

For those who might feel ambivalent about their present doctors, we have provided another questionnaire. We hope it helps you reflect on what to look for in your caregivers, and how to move ahead wisely in choosing the best doctors *for you*.

PRACTITIONER ASSESSMENT:
IS YOUR DOCTOR RIGHT FOR *YOU*?

1. Is your doctor courteous to you and supportive in general?
2. Does your doctor inspire you to want to do your best in relation to your health?
3. Is your doctor responsive and helpful with your anxieties, willing to answer your questions prior to procedures or prescriptions?
4. Does your doctor present very current research and valuable information (rather than seeming that he or she has been doing things the same way for many years without change)?

5. Does your doctor do a thorough job of physical, mental, emotional, and possibly even spiritual assessment in addition to relying on blood tests?

6. Is he or she willing to view you as an individual, perhaps with your own unique ranges of normal for certain tests?

7. Does your doctor generally present concerns about your health in a positive manner (one that avoids blaming you for your health problems and also avoids providing the scariest worst-case scenarios immediately)?

8. Does your doctor seem interested and act supportive when you mention vitamins or other natural protocols?

9. Will your doctor review materials you've brought in from your own research, such as a medical journal article or a respected health book?

10. Does your doctor view you as an equal partner in the health-care team?

11. Does your doctor answer your questions to your satisfaction, without leaving you feeling dismissed or brushed off?

12. Does your doctor ask about your wishes, preferences, and beliefs prior to coming up with a plan?

13. Will your doctor sign prescription slips to refer you to complementary practitioners of your choice?

14. Are the staff members in your doctor's office respectful and helpful? Is the environment conducive to healing?

15. Has your doctor been forthright and cooperative about your requests for ancillary treatments?

SCORING YOUR QUESTIONNAIRE

If you answered no to three or more of the above questions, we recommend that you consider "shopping" for a better match. For some people, including those who are especially sensitive, having even one no answer in the list above could be sufficient to warrant a reconsideration of your primary and related practitioners.

WHAT TO SHOW YOUR DOCTOR

Your medical practitioner may need some encouragement in order to become a full partner in diagnosing and treating your gland imbalance. You can facilitate this process by bringing to your appointment some compelling written material. Amid lecturing and providing telephone thyroid coaching related to our previous book, *Thyroid Power*, we have spoken with people from all over the country. They have generally relayed to us that alternative practitioners seem willing to look at books, magazine articles, newsletters, and especially references to the scientific literature.

Medical doctors, however, may be unmoved by anything except direct citations and articles from medical journals. Thus, you may want to show your practitioner only those items that will appeal to his or her preferred way of practicing, namely medical journal articles for MDs and practice-appropriate material for other health providers.

We have provided a sampling of articles and Web sites that can help you get started. Once you have shown your practitioner the journal article (properly highlighted regarding your specific needs), then ask if he or she can work with you to address these concerns.

We wish you good luck in finding the support and help you need.

IF YOU NEED ADDITIONAL HELP

If you cannot find a willing, knowledgeable practitioner, you may elect to have your tests interpreted by Drs. Richard or Karilee Shames in the context of a prepaid telephone coaching session. (See **www.FeelingFFF.com** or call toll-free (866) 468-4979 to schedule an appointment.)

If you are already working with a helpful practitioner, he or she would ideally place the lab order, or you can list your practitioner so that both of you would receive a copy of the results. If you require further support interpreting these results, a conference call can be arranged—or you or your practitioner can consult with Dr. Shames, faxing results to him and discussing their meaning to you in a prepaid telephone coaching session.

Some people who already have a practitioner consult with Dr. Shames to more fully understand their situation and to create the best possible plan. Some elect to have their local caregiver consult with Dr. Shames about their case. Others work with Karilee Shames on emotional issues and energy rebalancing maneuvers.

This new model of health education allows you to understand your metabolic and hormonal challenges while also assisting you in the process of making sensible decisions about how you might best proceed in achieving better hormonal health.

INDEX

ABOUT THE AUTHORS

Richard Shames, MD, is a graduate of Harvard University and the University of Pennsylvania Medical School. A founding member of the American Holistic Medical Association, he has served as adjunct faculty at UCSF Medical Center and Florida Atlantic University. He has been in private practice as a general practitioner for twenty-five years, currently at the Preventive Medicine Center in San Rafael, California, specializing in hormone treatment and in national personalized telephone hormone coaching via his Web sites www.FeelingFFF.com and www.thyroidpower.com. Dr. Shames is the coauthor of *Thyroid Power* (HarperCollins, 2001) with his wife, Karilee Shames, PhD, RN. Together they practice, lecture, and write extensively for health professionals and the general public on topics related to health promotion and integrative medicine.

Karilee Shames, PhD, RN, is a certified clinical specialist in psychiatric nursing and a certified holistic nurse. She served as an assistant professor of nursing at Florida Atlantic University from 1999 to 2002 and is currently in collaborative practice with Richard Shames, MD, specializing in providing emotional and spiritual healing for those challenged by gland imbalances. A low-thyroid person herself, Karilee copresents with Dr. Shames at health conferences nationwide, leads thyroid recovery groups, and also provides national telephone consultation for the mental, emotional, and spiritual aspects of these subtle gland conditions, helping patients to release distress, reclaim health, and make better life choices. Dr. Shames and her husband, Dr. Richard Shames, reside in the beautiful wine country of Northern California. Their three grown children are all currently in college or graduate programs.